W9-DFK-797

Bonita M. Veysey, PhD
Colleen Clark, PhD
Editors

Responding to Physical and Sexual Abuse in Women with Alcohol and Other Drug and Mental Disorders: Program Building

Responding to Physical and Sexual Abuse in Women with Alcohol and Other Drug and Mental Disorders: Program Building has been co-published simultaneously as *Alcoholism Treatment Quarterly*, Volume 22, Numbers 3/4 2004.

Pre-publication
REVIEWS,
COMMENTARIES,
EVALUATIONS . . .

"HIGHLY RECOMMENDED. Any clinician working with women (and their families) will appreciate the breadth and depth of this book and its use of clinical examples, treatment direction, and sobering statistics."

John Brick, PhD, MA, FAPA
Executive Director
Intoxicon International
Author of Drugs, the Brain and Behavior *and the* Handbook of the Medical Consequences of Alcohol and Drug Abuse

Responding to Physical and Sexual Abuse in Women with Alcohol and Other Drug and Mental Disorders: Program Building

Responding to Physical and Sexual Abuse in Women with Alcohol and Other Drug and Mental Disorders: Program Building has been co-published simultaneously as *Alcoholism Treatment Quarterly*, Volume 22, Numbers 3/4 2004.

The *Alcoholism Treatment Quarterly* Monographic "Separates"

Below is a list of "separates," which in serials librarianship means a special issue simultaneously published as a special journal issue or double-issue *and* as a "separate" hardbound monograph. (This is a format which we also call a "DocuSerial.")

"Separates" are published because specialized libraries or professionals may wish to purchase a specific thematic issue by itself in a format which can be separately cataloged and shelved, as opposed to purchasing the journal on an on-going basis.

"Separates" are carefully classified separately with the major book jobbers so that the journal tie-in can be noted on new book order slips to avoid duplicate purchasing.

You may wish to visit Haworth's website at . . .

http://www.HaworthPress.com

. . . to search our online catalog for complete tables of contents of these separates and related publications.

You may also call 1-800-HAWORTH (outside US/Canada: 607-722-5857), or Fax 1-800-895-0582 (outside US/Canada: 607-771-0012), or e-mail at:

docdelivery@haworthpress.com

Responding to Physical and Sexual Abuse in Women with Alcohol and Other Drug and Mental Disorders: Program Building, edited by Bonita M. Veysey, PhD. and Colleen Clark, PhD (Vol. 22, No. 3/4, 2004). *"Highly recommended. Any clinician working with women (and their families) will appreciate the breadth and depth of this book and its use of clinical examples, treatment direction, and sobering statistics." (John Brick, PhD, MA, FAPA, Executive Director, Intoxicon International; Author of Drugs, the Brain, and Behavior and the Handbook of the Medical Consequences of Alcohol and Drug Abuse)*

Alcohol Problems in the United States: Twenty Years of Treatment Perspective, edited by Thomas F. McGovern, EdD, and William L. White, MA (Vol. 20, No. 3/4, 2002). *An overview of trends in the treatment of alcohol problems over a 20-year period.*

Homelessness Prevention in Treatment of Substance Abuse and Mental Illness: Logic Models and Implementation of Eight American Projects, edited by Kendon J. Conrad, PhD, Michael D. Matters, PhD, Patricia Hanrahan, PhD, and Daniel J. Luchins, MD (Vol. 17, No. 1/2, 1999). *Provides you with new insights into how you can help your clients overcome political, economic, and environmental barriers to treatment that can lead to homelessness.*

Alcohol Use/Abuse Among Latinos: Issues and Examples of Culturally Competent Services, edited by Melvin Delgado, PhD (Vol. 16, No. 1/2, 1998). *"This book will have widespread appeal for practitioners and educators involved in direct service delivery, organizational planning, research, or policy development." (Steven Lozano Applewhite, PhD, Associate Professor, Graduate School of Social Work, University of Houston, Texas)*

Treatment of the Addictions: Applications of Outcome Research for Clinical Management, edited by Norman S. Miller, MD (Vol. 12, No. 2, 1994). *"Ambitious and informative. . . . Recommended to anybody involved in the practice of substance abuse treatment and research in treatment outcome." (The American Journal of Addictions)*

Self-Recovery: Treating Addictions Using Transcendental Meditation and Maharishi Ayur-Veda, edited by David F. O'Connell, PhD, and Charles N. Alexander, PhD (Vol. 11, No. 1/2/3/4, 1994). *"A scholarly trailblazer, a scientific first. . . . Those who work daily in the fight against substance abuse, violence, and illness will surely profit from reading this important volume. A valuable new tool in what may be America's most difficult battle." (Joseph Drew, PhD, Chair for Evaluation, Mayor's Advisory Committee on Drug Abuse, Washington, DC; Professor of Political Science, University of the District of Columbia)*

Treatment of the Chemically Dependent Homeless: Theory and Implementation in Fourteen American Projects, edited by Kendon J. Conrad, PhD, Cheryl I. Hultman, PhD, and John S. Lyons, PhD (Vol. 10, No. 3/4, 1993). *"A wealth of information and experience. . . . A very useful reference book for everyone seeking to develop their own treatment strategies with this patient group or the homeless mentally ill." (British Journal of Psychiatry)*

Treating Alcoholism and Drug Abuse Among Homeless Men and Women: Nine Community Demonstration Grants, edited by Milton Argeriou, PhD, and Dennis McCarty, PhD (Vol. 7, No. 1, 1990). *"Recommended to those in the process of trying to better serve chemically dependent homeless persons." (Journal of Psychoactive Drugs)*

Co-Dependency: Issues in Treatment and Recovery, edited by Bruce Carruth, PhD, and Warner Mendenhall, PhD (Vol. 6, No. 1, 1989). *"At last a book for clinicians that clearly defines co-dependency and gives helpful treatment approaches. Essential." (Margot Escott, MSW, Social Worker in Private Practice, Naples, Florida)*

The Treatment of Shame and Guilt in Alcoholism Counseling, edited by Ronald T. Potter-Efron, MSW, PhD, and Patricia S. Potter-Efron, MS, CACD III (Vol. 4, No. 2, 1989). *"Comprehensive in its coverage and provides important insights into the treatment of alcoholism, especially the importance to the recovery process of working through feelings of overwhelming shame and guilt. Recommended as required reading." (Australian Psychologist)*

Drunk Driving in America: Strategies and Approaches to Treatment, edited by Stephen K. Valle, ScD, CAC, FACATA (Vol. 3, No. 2, 1986). *Creative and thought-provoking methods related to research, policy, and treatment of the drunk driver.*

Alcohol Interventions: Historical and Sociocultural Approaches, edited by David L. Strug, PhD, S. Priyadarsini, PhD, and Merton M. Hyman (Supp. #1, 1986). *"A comprehensive and unique account of addictions treatment of centuries ago." (Federal Probation: A Journal of Correctional Philosophy)*

Treatment of Black Alcoholics, edited by Frances Larry Brisbane, PhD, MSW, and Maxine Womble, MA (Vol. 2, No. 3/4, 1985). *"Outstanding! In view of the paucity of research on the topic, this text presents some of the outstanding work done in this area." (Dr. Edward R. Smith, Department of Educational Psychology, University of Wisconsin-Milwaukee)*

Psychosocial Issues in the Treatment of Alcoholism, edited by David Cook, CSW, Christine Fewell, ACSW, and Shulamith Lala Ashenberg Straussner, DSW, CEAP (Vol. 2, No. 1, 1985). *"Well-written and informative; the topic areas are relevant to today's social issues and offer some new approaches to the treatment of alcoholics." (The American Journal of Occupational Therapy)*

Alcoholism and Sexual Dysfunction: Issues in Clinical Management, edited by David J. Powell, PhD (Vol. 1, No. 3, 1984). *"It does a good job of explicating the linkage between two of the most common health problems in the U.S. today." (Journal of Sex & Marital Therapy)*

Responding to Physical and Sexual Abuse in Women with Alcohol and Other Drug and Mental Disorders: Program Building

Bonita M. Veysey, PhD
Colleen Clark, PhD
Editors

Responding to Physical and Sexual Abuse in Women with Alcohol and Other Drug and Mental Disorders: Program Building has been co-published simultaneously as *Alcoholism Treatment Quarterly*, Volume 22, Numbers 3/4 2004.

The Haworth Press, Inc.

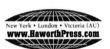

New York • London • Victoria (AU)
www.HaworthPress.com

Responding to Physical and Sexual Abuse in Women with Alcohol and Other Drug and Mental Disorders: Program Building has been co-published simultaneously as *Alcoholism Treatment Quarterly*, Volume 22, Numbers 3/4 2004.

The development, preparation, and publication of this work has been undertaken with great care. However, the publisher, employees, editors, and agents of The Haworth Press and all imprints of The Haworth Press, Inc., including The Haworth Medical Press® and Pharmaceutical Products Press®, are not responsible for any errors contained herein or for consequences that may ensue from use of materials or information contained in this work. Opinions expressed by the author(s) are not necessarily those of The Haworth Press, Inc. With regard to case studies, identities and circumstances of individuals discussed herein have been changed to protect confidentiality. Any resemblance to actual persons, living or dead, is entirely coincidental.

The Haworth Press, Inc., 10 Alice Street, Binghamton, 13904-1580 USA

Cover design by Kerry E. Mack

Library of Congress Cataloging-in-Publication Data

Responding to physical and sexual abuse in women with alcohol and other drug and mental disorders: program building / Bonita M. Veysey, Colleen Clark, editors.
  p. cm.
   "Co-published simultaneously as Alcoholism treatment quarterly, Volume 22, Numbers 3/4 2004."
  Includes bibliographical references and index.
  ISBN 0-7890-2603-1 (hard cover : alk. paper) – ISBN 0-7890-2604-X (soft cover : alk. paper)
  1. Abused women–Alcohol use. 2. Abused women–Drug use. 3. Abused women–Mental health.
  I. Veysey, Bonita M. II. Clark, Colleen. III. Alcoholism treatment quarterly.
HV6625.R47 2004
362.29´082–dc22

                     2004020036

Indexing, Abstracting & Website/Internet Coverage

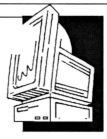

    This section provides you with a list of major indexing & abstracting services and other tools for bibliographic access. That is to say, each service began covering this periodical during the year noted in the right column. Most Websites which are listed below have indicated that they will either post, disseminate, compile, archive, cite or alert their own Website users with research-based content from this work. (This list is as current as the copyright date of this publication.)

Abstracting, Website/Indexing Coverage . . . . Year When Coverage Began

- *Abstracts in Anthropology* **1991**

- *Academic Abstracts/CD-ROM* **1995**

- *Academic Search Elite (EBSCO)* **1995**

- *Academic Search Premier (EBSCO)*
  <http://www.epnet.com/academic/acasearchprem.asp> **1995**

- *Addiction Abstracts is a quarterly journal published in*
  simultaneous print & online editions. This unique resource &
  reference tool is published in collaboration with the Natl
  Addiction Ctr & Carfax, Taylor & Francis
  <http://www.tandf.co.uk/addiction-abs> **1995**

- *Business Source Corporate: coverage of nearly 3,350 quality*
  magazines and journals; designed to meet the diverse
  information needs of corporations; EBSCO Publishing
  <http://www.epnet.com/corporate/bsourcecorp.asp> **1995**

- *Criminal Justice Abstracts* **1984**

- *EAP Abstracts Plus* **1995**

- *EBSCOhost Electronic Journals Service (EJS)*
  <http://ejournals.ebsco.com> **2001**

(continued)

- *EMBASE.com (The Power of EMBASE + MEDLINE Combined)*
  <http://www.embase.com> **1984**
- *EMBASE/Excerpta Medica Secondary Publishing Division.*
  Included in newsletters, review journals, major reference works,
  magazines & abstract journals <http://www.elsevier.nl> **1984**
- *Excerpta Medica . . . . See EMBASE* **1984**
- *e-psyche, LLC <http://www.e-psyche.net>* **2001**
- *Family & Society Studies Worldwide <http://www.nisc.com>* **1995**
- *Family Index Database <http://www.familyscholar.com>* **2003**
- *Health Source: Indexing & Abstracting of 160 selected*
  health related journals, updated monthly: EBSCO Publishing **1995**
- *Health Source Plus: Expanded version*
  of "Health Source": EBSCO Publishing **1995**
- *Index Guide to College Journals (core list compiled by integrating*
  48 indexes frequently used to support undergraduate programs
  in small to medium sized libraries) **1999**
- *Index to Periodical Articles Related to Law*
  <http://www.law.utexas.edu> **1984**
- *Lesbian Information Service*
  <http://www.lesbianinformationservice.org> **1992**
- *MasterFILE Elite: coverage of nearly 1,200 periodicals covering*
  general reference, business, health, education, general
  science, multi-cultural issues and much more; EBSCO
  Publishing <http://www.epnet.com/government/mfelite.asp> **1995**
- *MasterFILE Premier: coverage of more than 1,950 periodicals*
  covering general reference, business, health, education,
  general science, multi-cultural issues and much more;
  EBSCO Publishing
  <http://www.epnet.com/government/mfpremier.asp> **1995**
- *MasterFILE Select: coverage of nearly 770 periodicals covering*
  general reference, business, health, education, general science,
  multi-cultural issues and much more; EBSCO Publishing
  <http://www.epnet.com/government/mfselect.asp> **1995**
- *National Criminal Justice Reference Service <http://www.ncjrs.org>* **1998**
- *OCLC ArticleFirst <http://www.oclc.org/services/databases/>* **2003**
- *OCLC ContentsFirst <http://www.oclc.org/services/databases/>* **2003**
- *Psychological Abstracts (PsycINFO) <http://www.apa.org>* **1984**
- *Referativnyi Zhurnal (Abstracts Journal of the All-Russian*
  Institute of Scientific and Technical Information–in Russian) . . . **1984**

(continued)

- *Sexual Diversity Studies: Gay, Lesbian, Bisexual & Transgender Abstracts (Formerly Gay & Lesbian Abstracts) provides comprehensive & in-depth coverage of the world's GLBT literature compiled by NISC & published on the Internet & CD-ROM <http://www.nisc.com>*................ 2002

- *Social Services Abstracts <http://www.csa.com>* 1990

- *Social Work Abstracts <http://www.silverplatter.com/catalog/swab.htm>*............. 1991

- *SocioAbs <http://www.csa.com>*............................. 2003

- *Sociological Abstracts (SA) <http://www.csa.com>* 1990

- *Spanish Technical Information System on Drug Abuse Prevention "Sistema de Informacion Tecnica Sobre Prevention del Abuso de Drogas" (in Spanish) <http://www.idea-prevencion.com>* 1998

- *Studies on Women and Gender Abstracts <http://www.tandf.co.uk/swa>* 1989

- *SwetsWise <http://www.swets.com>* 2001

- *Violence and Abuse Abstracts: A Review of Current Literature on Interpersonal Violence (VAA)* 1995

- *zetoc <http://zetoc.mimas.ac.uk/>*........................... 2004

Special Bibliographic Notes related to special journal issues (separates) and indexing/abstracting:

- indexing/abstracting services in this list will also cover material in any "separate" that is co-published simultaneously with Haworth's special thematic journal issue or DocuSerial. Indexing/abstracting usually covers material at the article/chapter level.
- monographic co-editions are intended for either non-subscribers or libraries which intend to purchase a second copy for their circulating collections.
- monographic co-editions are reported to all jobbers/wholesalers/approval plans. The source journal is listed as the "series" to assist the prevention of duplicate purchasing in the same manner utilized for books-in-series.
- to facilitate user/access services all indexing/abstracting services are encouraged to utilize the co-indexing entry note indicated at the bottom of the first page of each article/chapter/contribution.
- this is intended to assist a library user of any reference tool (whether print, electronic, online, or CD-ROM) to locate the monographic version if the library has purchased this version but not a subscription to the source journal.
- individual articles/chapters in any Haworth publication are also available through the Haworth Document Delivery Service (HDDS).

Responding to Physical and Sexual Abuse in Women with Alcohol and Other Drug and Mental Disorders: Program Building

CONTENTS

Introduction   1
Bonita M. Veysey
Colleen Clark

Integration of Alcohol and Other Drug, Trauma and Mental
Health Services: An Experiment in Rural Services
Integration in Franklin County, MA   19
Bonita M. Veysey
Rene Andersen
Leslie Lewis
Mindy Mueller
Vanja M. K. Stenius

Creating Alcohol and Other Drug, Trauma, and Mental Health
Services for Women in Rural Florida: The Triad
Women's Project   41
Colleen Clark
Julienne Giard
Margo Fleisher-Bond
Sharon Slavin
Marion Becker
Arthur Cox

The Women Embracing Life and Living (WELL) Project:
Using the Relational Model to Develop Integrated
Systems of Care for Women with Alcohol/Drug Use
and Mental Health Disorders with Histories of Violence   63
Norma Finkelstein
Laurie S. Markoff

A Model for Changing Alcohol and Other Drug, Mental Health,
    and Trauma Services Practice: PROTOTYPES Systems
    Change Center   81
      Vivian B. Brown
      Elke Rechberger
      Paula Bjelajac

Boston Consortium of Services for Families in Recovery:
    A Trauma-Informed Intervention Model for Women's
    Alcohol and Drug Addiction Treatment   95
      Hortensia Amaro
      Sarah McGraw
      Mary Jo Larson
      Luz Lopez
      Rita Nieves
      Brenda Marshall

The Portal Project: A Layered Approach to Integrating Trauma
    into Alcohol and Other Drug Treatment for Women   121
      Sharon Cadiz
      Andrea Savage
      Diane Bonavota
      James Hollywood
      Erica Butters
      Michelle Neary
      Laura Quiros

New Directions for Families: A Family-Oriented Intervention
    for Women Affected by Alcoholism and Other Drug
    Abuse, Mental Illness and Trauma   141
      Nancy R. VanDeMark
      Ellen Brown
      Angela Bornemann
      Susan Williams

Allies: Integrating Women's Alcohol, Drug, Mental Health
    and Trauma Treatment in a County System   161
        Jennifer P. Heckman
        Frances A. Hutchins
        Jennifer C. Thom
        Lisa A. Russell

Integrated Trauma Services Teams for Women Survivors
    with Alcohol and Other Drug Problems and Co-Occurring
    Mental Disorders   181
        Roger D. Fallot
        Maxine Harris

Index   201

ABOUT THE EDITORS

Bonita M. Veysey, PhD, is Assistant Professor and Associate Dean for the School of Criminal Justice at Rutgers University-Newark. She is also the Director of the Center for Justice and Mental Health Research. Prior to her employment at Rutgers, Dr. Veysey was a Senior Research Associate at Policy Research Associates in Delmar, New York. During that time she was the Director of the Women's Program Core and the Associate Director of the National GAINS Center and the primary researcher in the area of mental health-criminal justice systems interactions. Dr. Veysey's research to date has focused on behavioral health and justice issues, including police interactions with persons with mental illnesses; psychiatric practices in jails and persons; diversion and treatment services for youth with behavioral health problems; and the effects of trauma. Dr. Veysey consults with local adult and juvenile justice agencies to help them respond to the needs of women and youth with histories of physical and sexual abuse.

Colleen Clark, PhD, is Research Assistant Professor in the Department of Mental Health, Law and Policy at the Louis de la Parte Florida Mental Health Institute, University of South Florida in Tampa. Dr. Clark is the Project Director and Principal Investigator from USF for three national collaborative mental health services research projects: (1) the Boley Homelessness Prevention Project, (2) the Triad Women's Project of the Women and Violence study, and (3) Manasota Homeless Families Project. She is the coordinator of the Florida Task Force on Trauma Services and a founding member of the National Trauma Consortium. She is a licensed clinical psychologist with a private practice in the Tampa area since 1989 and was associated for 10 years with Mental Health Care, Inc., a large urban community mental health center, both as Division Director and as a member of the Board of Directors. She is a longtime member of the Tampa Bay Association of Women Psychotherapists.

Introduction

Bonita M. Veysey, PhD
Colleen Clark, PhD

SUMMARY. The Women, Co-occurring Disorders and Violence Study is the first effort to address the significant lack of appropriate services for women with alcohol and other drug and mental health diagnoses who have experienced physical and/or sexual abuse. This program is sponsored by the Substance Abuse and Mental Health Services Administration's three Centers: the Center for Substance Abuse Treatment, the Center for Substance Abuse Prevention and the Center for Mental Health Services. The nine participating sites each developed a services

---

Bonita M. Veysey is affiliated with Rutgers-Newark, The State University of New Jersey, School of Criminal Justice. Colleen Clark is affiliated with the University of South Florida, Florida Mental Health Institute.

The authors would like to thank their SAMHSA Project Officers, Melissa Rael and Joanne Gampel of the Center for Substance Abuse Treatment; Susan Salasin and Kana Enomoto of the Center for Mental Health Services; and Jeanette Bevett-Mills of the Center for Substance Abuse Prevention. Without their dedication this project would not have been possible. The authors also would like to thank all of the women in their local communities who continue to bear witness to the strength of the human spirit.

The work described in this volume was funded under Guidance for Applicants (GFA) No. TI 00-003 entitled *Cooperative Agreement to Study Women with Alcohol, Drug Abuse and Mental Health (ADM) Disorders Who Have Histories of Violence: Phase II* from the Department of Health and Human Services, Public Health Service, Substance Abuse and Mental Health Services Administration's (SAMHSA) three centers: Center for Substance Abuse Treatment, Center for Mental Health Services and Center for Substance Abuse Prevention (March 2000).

[Haworth co-indexing entry note]: "Introduction." Veysey, Bonita M., and Colleen Clark. Co-published simultaneously in *Alcoholism Treatment Quarterly* (The Haworth Press, Inc.) Vol. 22, No. 3/4, 2004, pp. 1-18; and: *Responding to Physical and Sexual Abuse in Women with Alcohol and Other Drug and Mental Disorders: Program Building* (ed: Bonita M. Veysey, and Colleen Clark) The Haworth Press, Inc., 2004, pp. 1-18. Single or multiple copies of this article are available for a fee from The Haworth Document Delivery Service [1-800-HAWORTH, 9:00 a.m. - 5:00 p.m. (EST). E-mail address: docdelivery@haworthpress.com].

Digital Object Identifier: 10.1300/J020v22n03_01

1

integration intervention addressing the multiple needs of women with co-occurring disorders and histories of violence. As participants in a cross-site initiative, each site created their interventions within the guidelines established by a Federal Steering Committee. Under these guidelines, interventions must be gender-specific, culturally competent, trauma-informed and trauma-specific, comprehensive and integrated, and involve consumers/survivors/recovering persons (CSRs) in substantive and meaningful ways. In this work, each site describes their strategies for developing strategies for integrating services at two levels: at the clinical/individual level and at the services or system level. Within this framework, sites have created programs that are responsive to the strengths and needs of their own communities. *[Article copies available for a fee from The Haworth Document Delivery Service: 1-800-HAWORTH. E-mail address: <docdelivery@haworthpress.com> Website: <http://www.HaworthPress. com> © 2004 by The Haworth Press, Inc. All rights reserved.]*

KEYWORDS. Alcoholism, drug abuse, mental health, women, physical abuse, sexual abuse, services integration

Trauma is central in the lives of women with co-occurring alcohol and other drug (AOD) and mental health diagnoses. The prevalence of women within the psychiatric system with a history of interpersonal violence varies between 48-90% (Alexander, 1996; Jennings, 1997; Kalinowski & Penney, 1998; Mueser et al., 1998). A history of interpersonal violence among women with AOD disorders also is very common ranging from 55-99% (Jennings, 1997; Miller, 1994, 1996; Najavits et al., 1996). Further, a staggering 84% of extremely poor, housed women, and 92% of homeless women have experienced some form of severe physical or sexual violence during childhood and/or adulthood (Bassuk et al., 1996, 1998).

SERVICE SYSTEM ISSUES

Women with AOD and mental health diagnoses who have histories of physical and/or sexual abuse present unique challenges to service systems. Treatment systems serving women with co-occurring disorders generally are uncoordinated, fragmented, poorly organized or nonexistent (Blanch & Levin, 1998). Insurance reimbursement mechanisms and exclusionary criteria within the AOD and mental health treatment systems require each particular service setting to focus on narrowly defined, service-specific symptoms rather than addressing women in their wholeness and complexity. Lack of attention to the effects of trauma and their relationship to alcohol and drug use and mental health symptoms often leads to misdiagnosis and misdirected treatment focus, thus limiting the effectiveness of the intervention and sometimes causing harm (Carmen et al., 1996; Carmen & Rieker, 1989; Jennings, 1997; Kalinowski & Penny, 1998; Ridgley & van der Berg, 1997). Rarely are treatment services designed or adapted specifically for women thus limiting their accessibility, applicability and effectiveness (National Institute on Drug Abuse, 2002).

The individual and community cost of not addressing trauma and concomitant issues is staggering in terms of human, systems, and economic costs. When the underlying issue of trauma is not addressed, the physical, emotional and psychological manifestations of that trauma may persist and be expressed through addictions, somatic complaints, acute and chronic medical conditions, depression, and anxiety. Women often use expensive services, including emergency rooms, inpatient hospitalizations, respite facilities, or are remanded to the criminal justice system. Health care costs among patients who report childhood trauma (and in particular, child sexual abuse) are substantially increased (Walker et al., 1999). Treating only the symptoms of trauma, without addressing the trauma itself, carries the risk of increasingly severe and debilitating sequelae for the individual, and exhaustion of resources within the system providing care (Bassuk et al., 1998). In one study, cost of care for a woman with a history of sexual abuse was $10,888 greater than for a woman in the mental health system without a history of sexual abuse (Newman et al., 1998). Jennings (1994) estimates that over a 17-year period, the cost of care for her daughter, a survivor of childhood sexual abuse who was repeatedly misdiagnosed, mistreated, ignored, dismissed, and retraumatized within the mental health system, amounted to more than three million dollars. In addition, there is a lost potential for work and community contribution, as well as costs related to children, through the intergenerational impact of violence, involvement of child welfare services, legal costs, and out of home placements.

Federal Response

In the 1990s, emerging research literature was beginning to identify these major gaps in treatment responses, particularly the lack of services for persons with AOD and mental health disorders, persons with histories of childhood physical and sexual abuse, and women and other cultural groups. As a result, in 1998 the federal Substance Abuse and Mental Health Services Administration (SAMHSA) released a Guidance for Applicants to develop, implement and evaluate services for women with co-occurring disorders and histories of violence based on principles of integrated, gender-specific and trauma-informed care. The three SAMHSA centers, the Center for Substance Abuse Treatment, the Center for Substance Abuse Prevention and the Center for Mental Health Services, created a cooperative agreement to support local efforts to enhance, reconfigure or refine existing systems of care to address the specific needs of this population. The resulting "Women with Co-occurring Disorders and Violence Study's" primary goal is the generation and application of empirical knowledge about the development of an integrated systems approach, including the appropriate blend of services interventions, for the target populations of women and their children (Substance Abuse and Mental Health Services Administration, 1998).

To be eligible, applicants had to have at least two years demonstrated experience working in the field of women, alcohol and other drug abuse and mental health disorders and violence, and must be a part of a larger coalition of providers. The successful grantees ranged from city health networks, to consumer-led coalitions, to private, non-profit AOD treatment agencies.

In the first two years of the study these sites worked together within their communities and with the other study participants to develop integrated services to serve women with histories of abuse and co-occurring disorders as well as their children. This volume includes descriptions of nine sites' efforts to develop these services, the barriers and resources available in each service system, the resulting services, service systems and interventions, and lessons learned from the process.

LITERATURE REVIEW

Interpersonal violence in the lives of women and children is so prevalent as to be described as endemic in American society (Browne & Bassuk, 1997) and has gained recognition as a public health crisis of epidemic proportions (Alexander & Muenzenmaier, 1998; Bloom, 1995). The impact of this violence is profound, shattering trust and safety, fragmenting relationships and narrowing hope. Interpersonal violence, including physical and sexual assault, such as rape, incest, battering and murder, is so common for women, regardless of cultural affiliation and socioeconomic class, as to be described as a "normative" part of female experience in the United States today (Salasin & Rich, 1993). In fact, 20-30% of women in the general population report experiencing sexual and/or physical abuse during their lifetime (Commonwealth Fund, 1997; Mowbray et al., 1998). One million women report episodes of domestic violence each year in the U.S. (Manley, 1999). Women who were abused as children are at increased risk of rape and domestic violence as adults (Alexander & Muenzenmaier, 1998; Crowell & Burgess, 1996; Lipschitz et al., Sorkenn, 1996; Walker et al., 1999), and indeed, between 70-80% of women who have experienced domestic violence have also survived physical and/or sexual abuse during childhood (Manley, 1999). These numbers represent a low estimate of the prevalence of violence since the silencing that results from fear, shame, and stigma creates a gross underreporting of the numbers of women who have been traumatized (Alexander & Muenzenmaier, 1998; Commonwealth Fund, 1997). Additionally, women who have histories of abuse as adults or children are usually exposed to violence committed by intimates. Abuse is rarely a single event, but rather an ongoing nightmare.

Consequences of Violence

The violence that women experience has profound effects. Early childhood sexual and physical abuse rips at the core of an individual's developing sense of self, violating fundamental assumptions about the integrity and control of one's body and self. The world no longer appears to be safe, just and orderly (Carmen & Rieker, 1989; Herman, 1992; Prescott, 1998; Salasin, 1994). Women who experience physical and sexual abuse as children are at increased risk for depression (Bassuk et al., 1998; Commonwealth Fund, 1997, 1998; Miller, 1990, 1992, 1994, 1996); post-traumatic stress reactions (Bassuk et al., 1998; Commonwealth Fund, 1997, 1998; Haswell & Graham, 1996; Miller, 1996, 2000; Mueser et al., 1998; van der Kolk, 1996); suicidal ideations and attempts (Bassuk, Melnick & Browne, 1998; Dubo et al., 1997; Miller, 1996, 2000); poor self-esteem (Alexander & Muenzenmaier, 1998; Glover et al., 1996; Herman, 1992; Higgins, 1994); eating disorders (Herman, 1992; Janes, 1994; Miller, 1996, 2000); self-inflicted injury (Alexander & Muenzenmaier, 1998; Dallam, 1997; Haswell & Graham, 1996; Miller, 1996, 2000; Rea et al., 1997; Zlotnick et al., 1997); and chronic medical conditions such as pelvic pain, gastrointestinal problems, fibromyalgia, epilepsy, migraines, respiratory-related ailments, and cardiovascular problems in later life (Bassuk et al., 1998; Felitti et al., 1998; Green et al., 1997; Guidry, Miller & Daly, 2000; Miller, 1994, 1996; Reilly, 1997; van der Kolk, 1996).

Herman (1992) suggests that early childhood abuse leads to coping strategies, such as dissociation, unrealistic world views, splitting of personalities, suppressed affect, and hypervigilance that assist in a child's survival. As a child ages, he/she may engage in other behaviors meant to suppress feelings and memories directly related to earlier, or even current, abuse, including risk-taking (including sexual behavior and running away), self-injury, eating disorders, and alcohol and other drug use. This suggests that trauma is central and causally related to addiction and symptoms of traumatic stress, which are often misunderstood as symptoms of non-trauma-related mental illnesses (Alexander & Muenzenmaier, 1998; Amaro & Hardy-Fanta, 1995; Miller, 1996, 2000).

Many of the adaptive strategies women use to cope with physical and sexual violence ultimately work against them (Miller, 2000) causing them to be labeled and devalued and placing them at high risk for further sexual and physical violence (Alexander & Muenzenmaier, 1998; Bassuk et al., 1998; RachBeisel et al., 1999; Walker et al., 1999). Role loss resulting from labeling and involvement in the mental health and AOD systems is harmful to a woman's sense of self and consequent recovery (Alexander & Muenzenmaier, 1998; Mowbray et al., 1998). Women and their allies in homeless (Susko, 1991) and battered women's shelters (Warshaw, 1995), correctional systems (Galbraith, 1998; Veysey et al., 1998), substance recovery programs (Miller, 1994; Prescott, 1998), and psychiatric systems (Dare to Vision, 1995; Dende et al., 1997; Harris, 1997; Jennings, 1997; Prescott, 1998) testify in compelling detail about the negative impact of labeling and subsequent loss of credibility to bear witness to their own lives. As their credibility is challenged, the risk of loss expands to such areas as child custody (Stefan, 1998), autonomy, employment, and safety.

Research indicates that women who receive mental health, AOD and/or emergency medical services are rarely asked about the current level of danger they are experiencing or their prior histories of physical and sexual abuse (Browne, 1997; Carlson et al., 1997; Carmen et al., 1996; Commonwealth Fund, 1998; Harris et al., 1997; Levin & Blanch, 1998; Miller, 1996, 2000). Women who have been abused frequently are hesitant to reveal their histories, citing shame, embarrassment and hopelessness as the greatest deterrents to disclosure (Commonwealth Fund, 1998; Simmons et al., 1996). In addition, many have learned to minimize and pathologize their histories of violence, rather than seeking help to address the abuse, they present for specific "symptoms" instead (Harris, 1998). Of the few women whose abuse histories are known, only 10-20% report that their trauma has been adequately addressed in treatment (Alexander & Muenzenmaier, 1998).

There is an acute lack of trauma-informed, gender-specific, culturally competent care for women. Gender-specific responses require services to be sensitive to women's families, particularly their children. Children play a profoundly important role in a mother's recovery and sense of well-being (Bevett-Mills, 2000). However, existing mental health, rehabilitation and social services programs have largely ignored parenting as an important and valued role for women (Blanch et al., 1994). Women of color face even greater barriers to disclosure and access to services due to inherent racial biases that frequently misinterpret cultural cues and fail to protect them from future re-victimization. Neither hospital nor community-based interventions tend to treat people with regard for the gender, socioeconomic and cultural context in which they exist (Oyserman et al., 1994).

SAMHSA LEADERSHIP

In July of 1992, Public Law (P.L.) 102-321 created the Substance Abuse Mental Health Services Administration (SAMHSA) and its three constituent Centers, the Center for Substance Abuse Treatment (CSAT), the Center for Mental Health Services (CMHS) and the Center for Substance Abuse Prevention (CSAP). SAMHSA was established with a strong legislative mandate to support services for women and their children. Knowledge gained from CSAT's and CSAP's programs for women and children about the impact of violence, and from the CMHS program exploring the role of physical and sexual abuse in the lives of women with serious mental illness, raised serious concerns and questions about the complex interaction of violence, AOD and mental health disorders. As a result, there was a compelling need for a public health policy review that charted new directions in these areas (SAMHSA, 1998).

Under the earlier P.L. 102-141, the Office of Substance Abuse Prevention (currently the Center for Substance Abuse Prevention-CSAP) was authorized to provide support for demonstration projects allowing substance abusing women to live with their children in comprehensive residential prevention and treatment facilities with CSAP awarding 11 federal grants in September 1992. However, an amendment required CSAT to establish residential substance abuse treatment programs, leading CSAP to transfer these grants to CSAT in October 1992. CSAT administered and supported these residential substance abuse treatment programs for five years and in during time, twice (in 1993 and in 1995) awarded an additional 50 grants targeting pregnant and postpartum women, their infants and children, and women and children in residential treatment.

These programs pioneered new ground in the treatment of substance abusing women and their children and gained invaluable expertise and knowledge in the area. Those working in these programs realized that the women and children served were much more seriously traumatized by physical and sexual abuse than had been anticipated, and they began to restructure some of the services and treatment practices accordingly. In addition, a growing number of women were identified as having mental illnesses co-occurring with their alcohol and drug disorders.

Meanwhile in 1994, CMHS convened the "Dare to Vision" conference. It focused on the "second injury" caused by the lack of recognition, knowledge, and unresponsiveness to the effects of trauma by many providers. Consumer/survivor/recovering persons at this conference gave testimony to the all-encompassing and long-lasting impact of this "second injury."

It was through these focused initiatives and the knowledge gained from these programs that shaped the current initiative. This initiative promoted collaboration among the fields of AOD treatment and prevention, mental health treatment, and trauma in partnership with the consumer/survivor/recovering community to addressing the multiple needs of the women and their children whose lives had been impacted by violence/trauma, and the co-occurring disorders of AOD abuse and mental illness through an integrated, comprehensive service environment. This became the Women, Co-Occurring Disorders and Violence Study (WCDVS), a five-year initiative jointly supported by the three centers of SAMHSA.

STUDY DESCRIPTION

The primary goal of the Women and Violence Study is the generation and application of empirical knowledge about the development of an integrated systems approach, and the effectiveness of this approach, including the appropriate blend of services interventions, for women with

AOD and mental health disorders and histories of violence and their children. This two-phase study is designed to measure individual-level and systems changes during and after the course of the services interventions provided to women and their children. Knowledge that is gained from this SAMHSA study is expected to be useful in advancing national, state and local policy that affects how the various systems of care respond to women with co-occurring disorders who have histories of violence.

Target Population

The target population is comprised of women, aged 18 and older, with experience of physical and/or sexual abuse who meet the diagnostic criteria for: (1) DSM-IV Axis I substance-related disorder (excluding caffeine and nicotine-related disorders); and (2) who meet the criteria for DSM-IV Axis I mental disorder or Axis II personality disorder. Either the AOD-related disorder or the mental health/personality disorder must be current (within the past 30 days) while the other disorder must have occurred within the past five years. In addition, the woman must have had at least two distinct treatment or service episodes within the mental health, AOD, or other system (e.g., criminal justice) that provides AOD/mental health care.

Phase One Goal and Objectives

The goal of Phase One was the development and implementation of integrated systems of care for women with co-occurring disorders who are victims of violence, and for their children. Within this goal, the objectives included: (1) the documentation of the integration strategies across participating sites through a qualitative evaluation; (2) the design of guidance and minimum requirements of services intervention models that would be fully implemented in Phase Two; and (3) the development of the cross-site outcome evaluation and protocols for use in Phase Two (SAMHSA, 1998).

Phase Two Goal and Objectives

The primary goal of this phase of the study was to test the effectiveness of integrated strategies and service intervention models for the target population of women. This goal was accomplished through a multi-model intervention study with quasi-experimental (non-random) comparison groups using a common interview protocol at baseline, 6 months, and 12 months.

The objectives of this phase were: (1) document and compare models for providing services to women with co-occurring disorders and histories of violence; (2) identify and measure the relationships between components of the integrated services and document the strategies used to achieve services integration; (3) measure the effectiveness of these innovative service models as compared to one another and to services as usual on outcomes for individuals and participating organizations; (4) examine specific factors within these integrated service models, such as trauma treatment approaches, CSR integration, costs, parenting interventions, and cultural or other subgroup variations and their impact on observed outcomes; and (5) synthesize lessons learned regarding models of services provision, strategies for services integration, innovative accomplishments regarding factors within integrated service models, and summarize local, state, and national public policy impacts that are project-related.

Phase I Activities

Prior to Phase II funding, each site had to demonstrate that the services in the integrated condition were integrated, comprehensive, trauma-informed, gender-specific, and involved CSRs in meaningful ways. During Phase I, the Steering Committee voted that, for the Integrated Condition, each site must demonstrate that they are operating at or above the third level of service system integration (i.e., coordination). Services integration at the coordination level is a process by which two or more agencies, service providers or community groups establish linkages to share information, resources, funding, and policy development. Commonly, written memoranda of understanding and other inter-agency agreements are implemented and guide the activities. Regular meetings of agency administrators, clinical staff, representatives of the community groups and the women served occur along with cross-training and sharing of resources. Activities are shared while agencies remain autonomous, and programs work together with common goals or outcomes. The major focus is on the relationships among the core service providers who contribute to the full array of comprehensive and integrated services being provided to women and children. It is conceptualized at two levels: (1) organizational and (2) clinical. Both levels must be achieved to expect improved participant outcomes. At the organizational level, services integration focuses on the linkages developed between a core lead agency or set of agencies and the full array of other agencies/programs that need to be involved in order for an intervention model to be considered comprehensive for the women and their children. At the clinical level, services integration focuses on the content of service delivery and the ways in which mental health, AOD, and trauma interventions are combined in a concurrent manner to enhance client outcomes.

Each study site participating in Phase II also was required to demonstrate that their Integrated Services condition had at least those service providers and support systems necessary to offer all of the core services as members of the "broad array of service providers and support systems" including: outreach and engagement; screening and assessment; treatment activities; parenting skills; resource coordination and advocacy; trauma-specific services; crisis intervention; and peer-run services.

SAMHSA is committed to services that effectively meet the critical needs of individuals and families of the nation's diverse populations who are impacted by, or at risk for, AOD and mental health problems. In keeping with this commitment, all prevention and treatment services must address gender, age, development, racial, ethnic and cultural issues, and related factors such as geographic localities and economic environments. Additionally, SAMHSA believes that, because families and consumers/recovering persons contribute significantly to knowledge development, they must be appropriately involved in all levels of problem definition, program planning, implementation, and evaluation of SAMHSA projects. Therefore, SAMHSA is committed to funding projects that are culturally competent, gender-specific, age appropriate, and customer driven (family, consumer/recovering person, and community) in their approaches.

OVERVIEW OF VOLUME

In this volume, authors from a wide variety of settings discuss the processes by which their programs and service systems were transformed in response to the needs of women with alcohol and other drug use disorders, mental health diagnoses, and histories of interpersonal violence who have been high utilizers of behavioral healthcare services. Interventions ranging from the clinical and individual level to large systems level innovations are described in detail as well as strategies for adapting them to a variety of "real world" situations.

In the four opening chapters, two sites describe the challenges faced in rural or semi-rural settings and two discuss large system interventions in major urban centers. Veysey et al. describe a collaboration between mental health and domestic violence service providers serving women in rural Massachusetts. This project is unique in that the entire project has been developed and managed by women who are consumers/survivors/recovering persons (CSRs) themselves. Three women's drop-in centers serve as the focal point of the intervention and offer coordinated trauma, AOD and mental health support, trauma recovery groups, coordinated referral and peer resource advocacy. Clark et al. come from a more traditional service setting, but are also operating in rural and semi-rural areas, in this case central Florida. They describe the strategies used to develop collaborations among AOD treatment programs, mental health centers, CSRs and others to successfully develop interventions with a trauma focus effectively delivered in this community.

The Cambridge, Massachusetts, site (Finkelstein et al.) developed integration strategies at the state level. Three dually licensed AOD and mental health providers collaborated to provide integrated interventions grounded in gender specific theory valuing women's roles and relations. They describe such strategies as Memoranda of Understanding (MOUs), cross-referrals, information sharing, interagency service planning, resource coordination councils, and the role of the State Leadership Council in developing relevant policies and pilot projects. On the west coast, a large multi-services agency providing residential, outpatient and day treatment services for alcohol or other substance abuse, mental health, HIV/AIDS, and domestic violence to women and children in Los Angeles County is the lead agency (Brown et al.). The roles and functions of interagency coordinating bodies in forming a responsive system are presented in detail.

The next four chapters expand these concepts. Two chapters emphasize culturally competent services for women of color. In Boston, Amaro et al. base their interventions in a city health department. They describe an integrated system of services housed within three AOD treatment modalities; outpatient counseling, methadone maintenance and residential treatment; serving primarily Latina and African American women in metropolitan Boston. An emphasis on providers of diverse backgrounds and bicultural and bilingual program materials is evident throughout all program elements. Similarly, Cadiz et al. write of a New York City based program which serves primarily African-American and Latina women with an emphasis on cultural awareness and sensitivity. Their interventions are provided within a large multi-service agency with residential and outpatient AOD abuse and mental health services, and a layering strategy is used to enhance trauma treatment.

Metropolitan Denver is the setting for the services described by VanDeMark et al., with an emphasis on supporting healthy families. A comprehensive residential and outpatient treatment program provides up to four months of intensive residential treatment to women and their children including trauma-specific services, a domestic violence group, parenting skills, treatment for co-occurring disorders, and comprehensive employment services. Four-month outpatient continuing care follows residential treatment. A program in northern California is as an example of yet another organizational level (Heckman et al.). A small county provider of health care services for people with AOD and mental health utilizes a Primary Treatment Network of five AOD treatment programs.

In the final chapter, although historically focused on persons with psychiatric disorders, the District of Columbia (Fallot et al.) trauma collaboration has a long history of recognizing and responding to the important issues of co-occurring AOD and mental health disorders and the impact of trauma on the lives of women they serve. This chapter emphasizes the importance of the full integration of CSRs and describes strategies to inform services at all levels about the impact of trauma.

Many similarities exist among these nine sites and, at the same time, each service system reflects the social and historical environment in which it is embedded. The strength of the SAMHSA initiative lies in both the similarities and differences. It is hoped that these nine sites' descriptions based upon the five years of experience in developing, implementing and evaluating integrated services for women with AOD and mental health disorders who have histories of physical and/or sexual abuse will aid communities in developing their own services for women with similar problems.

REFERENCES

Alexander, M.J. (1996). Women with co-occurring addictive and mental disorders: An emerging profile of vulnerability. *American Journal of Orthopsychiatry, 66,* 61-70.
Alexander M.J. & Muenzenmaier, K. (1998). Trauma, addiction and recovery: Addressing public health epidemics among women with severe mental illness. In B.L. Levin, A.

Blanch, and A. Jennings (Eds.), *Women's Mental Health Services: A Public Health Perspective* (pp. 215-39). Thousand Oaks, CA: Sage Publications.

Amaro, H., & Hardy-Fanta, C. (1995). Gender relations in addiction and recovery. *Journal of Psychoactive Drugs, 27*(4), 325-327.

Bassuk, E.L. Weinreb, L.F., Buckner, J.C., Browne, A., Salomon, A., & Bassuk, S. (1996). The characteristics and needs of sheltered homeless and low income housed mothers. *JAMA, 276*(8), 640-646.

Bassuk, E.L., Melnick, S., & Browne, A. (1998). Responding to the needs of low-income and homeless women who are survivors of family violence. *Journal of the American Medical Women's Association, 53*, 57-64.

Bassuk, E.L., Perloff, J., & Garcia Coll, C. (1998). The plight of extremely poor Puerto-Rican and non-hispanic white single mothers. *Social Psychiatry and Psychiatric Epidemiology, 33*, 326-336.

Bevett-Mills, J. (2000). Quote from the following article by Barton, J.: Violence against women: SAMHSA's response. *SAMHSA News, 8*(4), 5-8.

Blanch, A.K., & Levin, B.L. (1998). Organization and services delivery. In B.L.Levin., and A.K. Blanch (Eds.), *Women's Mental Health Services: A Public Health Perspective* (pp. 5-18). Thousand Oaks, CA: Sage Publications.

Blanch, A.K., Nicholson, J., & Purcell, J. (1994). Parents with severe mental illness and their children: The need for human services integration. *Journal of Mental Health Administration, 21*(4), 388-396.

Bloom, S.L. (1995). The germ theory of trauma: The impossibility of ethical neutrality. In B.H. Stamm (Ed.), *Secondary Traumatic Stress: Self-Care Issues for Clinicians, Researchers and Educators* (pp. 257-276). Lutherville, MD: Sidran.

Browne, A. & Bassuk, S. (1997). Intimate violence in the lives of homeless and poor housed women: Prevalence and patterns in an ethnically diverse sample. *American Journal of Orthopsychiatry, 67*, 261-278.

Carlson, E.B, Furby, L., Armstrong, J., & Shlaes, J. (1997). A conceptual framework for the long-term psychological effects of traumatic childhood abuse. *Child Maltreatment: Journal of the American Professional Society on the Abuse of Children, 2*(3), 272-295.

Carmen, E.H., Crane, B., Dunnicliff, M., Holochuck, S., Prescott, L., Rieker, P.P., Stefan, S., & Stromberg, N. (1996). *Massachusetts Department of Mental Health Task Force on the Restraint and Seclusion of Persons Who Have Been Physically or Sexually Abused: Report and Recommendations.* Boston, MA: Department of Mental Health.

Carmen, E.H. & Rieker, P.P. (1989) A psychosocial model of the victim-to-patient process: Implications for treatment. *Psychiatric Clinics of North America, 12*, 431-443.

Commonwealth Fund. (1997). *Facts on Abuse and Violence: The Commonwealth Fund Survey of the Health of Adolescent Girls.* New York: Louis Harris and Associates, Inc.

Commonwealth Fund. (1998). *Addressing Domestic Violence and Its Consequences.* New York: Louis Harris and Associates, Inc.

Crowell, N.A. & Burgess, A.W. (1996). Understanding violence against women. National Research Council, Commission on Behavioral and Social Sciences and Education, Committee on Law and Justice, Panel on Research on Violence Against Women, Washington, DC: National Academy Press.

Dallam, S.J. (1997). The identification and management of self-mutilating patients in primary care. *The Nurse Practitioner, 22*(5), 151-153, 159-65.

Dare to Vision: Shaping the National Agenda for Women, Abuse and Mental Health Services. Proceedings of a Conference held July 14-16, 1994 in Arlington, VA, co-sponsored by the Center for Mental Health Services and Human Resource Association of the Northeast, (1995). Holyoke, MA: Human Resource Association.

Dende, J.D., Duca, C., Hobbs, M., & Landis, C.L. (1997). As told to . . . In M. Harris and C.L. Landis (Eds.), *Sexual Abuse in the Lives of Women Diagnosed with Serious Mental Illness* (pp. 181-215). Netherlands: Harwood Academic Publishers.

Dubo, E.D., Zanarini, M.C., Lewis, R.E., & Williams, A.A. (1997). Childhood antecedents of self-destructiveness in borderline personality disorder. *Canadian Journal of Psychiatry, 42*(1), 63-69.

Felitti, V.J, Anda, R.F., Nordenberg, D., Williamson, D.F., Spitz, A.M., Edwards, V., Koss, M.P., & Marks, J.S. (1998). Relationship of childhood abuse and household dysfunction to many of the leading causes of death in adults. *American Journal of Preventative Medicine, 14*, 245-258.

Galbraith, S. (1998). *And So I Began to Listen to Their Stories . . . Working with Women in the Criminal Justice System.* Delmar, NY: National GAINS Center for People with Co-Occurring Disorders in the Justice System.

Glover, N.M., Janikowski, T.P., & Benshoff, J.J. (1996). Substance abuse and past incest contact: A national perspective. *Journal of Substance Abuse Treatment, 13*(3), 185-193.

Green, B.L., Epstein, S.A., Krupnick, J.L., & Rowland, J.H. (1997). Trauma and medical illness: Assessing trauma-related disorders in medical settings. In J.P. Wilson and T.M. Keane (Eds.), *Assessing Psychological Trauma and PTSD* (pp. 160-191). New York, NY: The Guilford Press.

Harris, M. & Landis, C.L. (Eds.) (1997). *Sexual Abuse in the Lives of Women Diagnosed with Serious Mental Illness.* Netherlands: Harwood Academic Publishers.

Harris, M. (1998). *Trauma Recovery and Empowerment: A Clinician's Guide to Working with Women in Groups.* New York: Free Press.

Harvey, M. (1996). An ecological view of psychological trauma and trauma recovery. *Journal of Traumatic Stress, 9*, 3-23.

Haswell, D.E. & Graham, M. (1996). Self-inflicted injuries: Challenging knowledge, skills and compassion. *Canadian Family Physician, 42*, 1756-58, 1761-64.

Herman, J.L. (1992). *Trauma and Recovery: The Aftermath of Violence-From Domestic Abuse to Political Terror.* New York: Basic Books.

Higgins, G.O. (1994). *Resilient Adults: Overcoming a Cruel Past.* San Francisco, CA: Jossey-Bass.

Janes, J. (1994). Their own worst enemy? Management and prevention of self-harm. *Professional Nursing, 9*(12), 838-841.

Jennings, A. (1994). On being invisible in the mental health system. *Journal of Mental Health Administration, 21*(4), 374-387.

Jennings, A. (1997). On being invisible in the mental health system. In M. Harris and C. Landis (Eds.), *Sexual Abuse in the Lives of Women Diagnosed with Serious Mental Illness* (pp. 162-180). Netherlands: Harwood Academic Publishers.

Kalinowski, C. & Penney, D. (1998). Empowerment and women's mental health services. In B. Levin, A. Blanch and A. Jennings (Eds.), *Women's Mental Health Services: A Public Health Perspective*. Thousand Oaks, CA: Sage Publications, Inc.

Lebowitz, L., Harvey, M.R., & Herman, J.L. (1993). A stage-by-dimension model of recovery from sexual trauma. *Journal of Interpersonal Violence, 8*(3), 378-391.

Levin, B.L. & Blanch, A.K. (Eds.) (1998). *Women's Mental Health Services: A Public Health Perspective*. Thousand Oaks, CA: Sage Publications.

Lipschitz, D.S., Kaplan, M.L., Sorkenn, J.B., Paedda, G.L., Chorney, P., & Asnis, G.M. (1996). Prevalence and characteristics of physical and sexual abuse among psychiatric outpatients. *Psychiatric Services, 47*(2), 189-191.

Manley, J.O. (1999). Battered women and their children: A public policy response. *Affilia, 14*(4), 439-459.

Miller, A. (1990). *Banished Knowledge: Facing Childhood Injuries*. New York: Doubleday.

Miller, D. (1994). *Women Who Hurt Themselves*. New York: Basic Books.

Miller, D. (1996). Challenging self-harm through transformation of the trauma story. *Sexual Addiction and Compulsivity, 3*(3), 213-227.

Miller, D. & Guidry, L. (2001). *Addictions and Trauma Recovery: Healing the Body, Mind and Spirit*. New York: W.W. Norton.

Mowbray, C.T., Oyserman, D., Saunders, D., & Rueda-Riedle, A. (1998). Women with sever mental disorders: Issues and service needs. In B.L. Levin and A.K. Blanch (Eds.), *Women's Mental Health Services: A Public Health Perspective* (pp. 175-200). Thousand Oaks, CA: Sage Publications, Inc.

Mueser, K.T., Goodman, L.B., Trumbetta, S.L., Rosenberg, S.D., Osher, F.C., Vidaver, R., Auciello, P., & Foy, D.W. (1998). Trauma and posttraumatic stress disorder in severe mental illness. *Journal of Counseling and Clinical Psychology, 66*(3), 493-499.

Najavits, L.M., Weiss, R.D., & Liese, B.S. (1996). Group cognitive behavioral therapy for women with PTSD and substance use disorder. *Journal of Substance Abuse Treatment, 13*(1), 13-22.

National Center for Service Integration. (1994). "Providing Comprehensive Integrated Services for Children and Families: Why Is It so Hard?" *NCSI News*, Winter: 1-3.

National Institute on Drug Abuse. *NIDA Notes: Articles That Address Women and Gender Differences Research*. Rockville, MD: Department of Health and Human Services.

Newman, D.L., Moffitt, T.E., Caspi, A., & Silva, P.A. (1998). Comorbid mental disorders: Implications for treatment and sample selection. *Journal of Abnormal Psychology, 107*(2), 305-311.

Oyserman, D., Mowbray, C.T., & Zemencuk, J.K. (1994). Resources and supports for mothers with severe mental illness. *Health and Social Work, 19*(2), 132-141.

Prescott, L. (1998). *Women Emerging in the Wake of Violence*. Culver City, CA: Prototypes Systems Change Center.

RachBeisel, J., Scott, J., & Dixon, L. (1999). Co-occurring severe mental illness and substance use disorders: A review of recent research. *Psychiatric Services, 50*(11), 1427-1434.

Rea, K., Aiken, F., & Borastero, C. (1997). Building therapeutic staff: Client relationship with women who self-harm. *Women's Health Issues, 7*(2), 121-125.

Ridgley, S. & van der Berg, P. (1997). *Women and Coercion in Mental Health Treatment: Commitment, Involuntary Medication, Seclusion & Restraint*. Tampa, Florida: Louis de la Parte Mental Health Institute, Department of Mental Health Law and Policy.

Salasin, S.E. & Rich, R.F. (1993). Mental health policy for victims of violence: The case against women. In J.P. Wilson and B. Raphael (Eds.), *International Handbook of Traumatic Stress Syndromes* (pp. 947-955). New York: Plenum Press.

Simmons, K.P., Sack, T., & Miller, G. (1996). Sexual abuse and chemical dependency: Implications for women in recovery. *Women & Therapy, 19*(2), 17-30.

Stefan, S. (1998). The impact of law on women with diagnoses of borderline personality disorder related to childhood sexual abuse. In B. Levin, A. Blanch and A. Jennings (Eds.), *Women's Mental Health Services: A Public Health Perspective*. Thousand Oaks, CA: Sage Publications.

Substance Abuse and Mental Health Services Administration. (1998). *Cooperative Agreement to Study Women with Alcohol, Drug Abuse & Mental Health (ADM) Disorders Who Have Histories of Violence. Washington, DC, May 1998* (Catalog of Federal Domestic Assistance No. 93.230). Guidance for Applicants (GFA) No. TI 98-004. Washington, DC: SAMHSA.

Susko, M.A. (Ed.) (1991). *Cry of the Invisible: Writings from the Homeless and Survivors of Psychiatric Hospitals*. Baltimore and Montreal: Conservatory Press.

Talbott, J.A. (1995). Evaluation the Johnson Foundation program on chronic mental illness: An interview with Howard Goldman. *Psychiatric Services, 45*(5), 501-503.

van der Kolk, B.A. (1996). The body keeps the score: Approaches to the psychobiology of posttraumatic stress disorder. In B.A. van der Kolk, A.C. McFarlane and L. Weisaeth (Eds.), *Traumatic Stress: The Effects of Overwhelming Experience on Mind, Body and Society* (pp. 303-327). New York: The Guilford Press.

van der Kolk, B.A. (1996). The complexity of adaptation to trauma: Self-regulation, stimulus discrimination, and characterological development. In B.A. van der Kolk, A.C. McFarlane and L. Weisaeth (Eds.), *Traumatic Stress: The Effects of Overwhelming Experience on Mind, Body and Society* (pp. 182-213). New York: The Guilford Press.

Veysey, B.M. (1997). Specific needs of women diagnosed with mental illness in U.S. jails. In B.L. Levin, and A.K. Blanch's (Eds.), *Women's Mental Health Services: A Public Health Perspective* (pp. 368-89). Thousand Oaks, CA: Sage Publications.

Veysey, B.M., De Cou, K., & Prescott, L. (1998). Effective management of female jail detainees with histories of physical and sexual abuse. *American Jails, 12*(2): 50-54.

Walker, E.A., Unutzer, J., Rutter, C., Gelfand, A., Saunders, K., VonKorff, M., Koss, M.P., & Katon, W. (1999). Cost of health care used by women HMO members with a history of childhood abuse and neglect. *Archives of Psychiatry, 56*, 609-613.

Walker, E.A., Gelfand, A., Katon, W.J., Koss, M.P., Von Korff, M., Bernstein, D., & Russo, J. (1999). Adult health status of women with histories of childhood abuse and neglect. *American Journal of Medicine, 107*, 332-339.

Warshaw, C. (1995). Violence and women's health: Old models, new challenges. *Dare to Vision: Shaping the National Agenda for Women, Abuse and Mental Health Services: Proceedings of a Conference held July 14-16, 1994 in Arlington VA, co-spon-*

sored by the Center for Mental Health Services and Human Association of the Northeast. Holyoke, MA: Human Resource Association.

Yessian, M.R. (1995). Learning from experience: Integrating human services. *Public Welfare*, Summer, 34-42.

Zlotnick, C., Shea, M.T., Recupero, P., Bidadi, K., Pearlstein, T., & Brown, P. (1997). Trauma, dissociation, impulsivity, and self-mutilation among substance abuse patients. *American Journal of Orthopsychiatry, 67*(4), 650-54.

Integration of Alcohol and Other Drug, Trauma and Mental Health Services: An Experiment in Rural Services Integration in Franklin County, MA

Bonita M. Veysey, PhD
Rene Andersen, MSW
Leslie Lewis, MA
Mindy Mueller, PhD
Vanja M. K. Stenius, MA

SUMMARY. The Franklin County Women's Research Project is a collaboration among the Western Massachusetts Training Consortium, the Franklin Medical Center, three Women's Resource Centers located across the county, and local consumer/survivor/recovering women (CSRs). This project is unusual in two ways: (1) it is a rural site, and (2) the project was

Bonita M. Veysey is affiliated with Rutgers-Newark, The State University of New Jersey, School of Criminal Justice. Rene Andersen, Leslie Lewis, and Mindy Mueller are affiliated with Western Massachusetts Training Consortium. Vanja M. K. Stenius is affiliated with Rutgers-Newark, The State University of New Jersey, School of Criminal Justice.

The authors wish to thank all of the Franklin County community–the courageous women, resource center volunteers and staff persons, hospital and service providers, and concerned citizens–for their support and belief in this important work.

The Franklin County Women's Research Project is funded by the Substance Abuse and Mental Health Services Administration (Grant #93-230).

[Haworth co-indexing entry note]: "Integration of Alcohol and Other Drug, Trauma and Mental Health Services: An Experiment in Rural Services Integration in Franklin County, MA." Veysey, Bonita M. et al. Co-published simultaneously in *Alcoholism Treatment Quarterly* (The Haworth Press, Inc.) Vol. 22, No. 3/4, 2004, pp. 19-39; and: *Responding to Physical and Sexual Abuse in Women with Alcohol and Other Drug and Mental Disorders: Program Building* (ed: Bonita M. Veysey, and Colleen Clark) The Haworth Press, Inc., 2004, pp. 19-39. Single or multiple copies of this article are available for a fee from The Haworth Document Delivery Service [1-800-HAWORTH, 9:00 a.m. - 5:00 p.m. (EST). E-mail address: docdelivery@haworthpress.com].

designed, implemented and evaluated by CSRs. The program model integrates services at the person level and at the system level. The Women's Resource Centers are the focal points for the individual level services integration offering women support through their peers, including AA/NA meetings, trauma recovery groups using the Addiction and Trauma Recovery Model (ATRIUM), Peer Resource Advocates, writing, art, and body awareness programs, and a variety of opportunities. The guiding principle is that women heal when they find the resources within themselves to define their lives and engage in activities and work that is meaningful to them. These Centers work in conjunction with the formal treatment systems. Services integration is accomplished through the Services Integration Committee comprised of the mental health, AOD and domestic violence providers, the Community Coordination Council comprised of a wider network of service and support providers, and through the activities of the Trauma Liaison, an employee of Franklin Medical Center who chairs the committees and provides consultation on women with trauma histories. *[Article copies available for a fee from The Haworth Document Delivery Service: 1-800-HAWORTH. E-mail address: <docdelivery@haworthpress.com> Website: <http://www.HaworthPress.com> © 2004 by The Haworth Press, Inc. All rights reserved.]*

KEYWORDS. Alcoholism, drug abuse, women, physical abuse, sexual abuse, services integration, rural

INTRODUCTION

Women with co-occurring alcohol and other drug (AOD) and mental health disorders and histories of violence present unique challenges to service providers who are often ill equipped to adequately deal with the multiple issues in these women's lives and are seldom aware of the women's trauma histories (Miller, 1996; Miller & Guidry, 2001; Commonwealth Fund, 1997; Levin & Blanch, 1998; Browne & Bassuk, 1997; Carlson et al., 1997; Harris & Landis, 1997; Carmen et al., 1996). Services are generally fragmented, poorly organized or nonexistent (Blanch & Levin, 1998). When available, services are often insensitive to gender, culture or socioeconomic context (Oyserman et al., 1994) and rarely address trauma adequately (Alexander & Muenzenmaier, 1998). In addition, exclusionary practices within the AOD and mental health treatment systems fragment women's care as each service setting focuses on narrowly defined, service-specific symptoms rather than addressing women in their wholeness and complexity. For women with the three tightly interconnected problems of trauma, AOD and mental health disorders, services should be gender-specific (Bevett-Mills, 2000; Blanch et al., 1994), trauma-specific (Miller, 1990, 1994, 1996; Miller & Guidry, 2001; Harris, 1994, 1998; Harvey, 1991), culturally sensitive (Oysterman et al., 1994), multidisciplinary, comprehensive, and coordinated to address the broad range of their needs (Alexander & Muenzenmaier, 1998).

The Franklin County Women and Violence Project (FCWVP) is an innovative community-based intervention for women with histories of trauma and co-occurring AOD and mental health disorders living in a rural community that attempts to address the deficiencies in the existing service system through individual- and systems-level service integration strategies. As part of a national study implementing and evaluating interventions for women who have been victims of violence and have co-occurring disorders the FCWVP has facilitated changes in traditional service delivery in Franklin County as well as initiated new services using a Consumer/Survivor/Recovering Person (CSR), or peer-driven, model. The FCWVP is unique within the national study in that it is one of two rural sites and the only site that is predominantly designed, implemented and operated by CSRs. This is significant for two reasons. First, rural service development traditionally has been difficult. Second, while different aspects of the FCWVP project have been studied individually (e.g., strength-based empowerment model, asset-based community development, peer-run model), this intervention is grounded in an integrated gender-specific, human development theory that encompasses all of these components. The intervention explicitly links theoretical constructs of recovery and growth with specific services and supports. This involves two components: (a) as a gender-specific human growth model, the FCWVP offers a unique opportunity to investigate the relationship between symptom reduction and "wellness," and (b) as a CSR-driven model, the FCWVP offers the opportunity to contrast professional-delivered services with peer-delivered supports.

OVERVIEW

Systems and Services Integration

Studies of services and systems integration demonstrate that integrated *systems* reduce redundancy and costs, but have little direct effect on persons receiving services (Morrissey et al., 1993; Talbott, 1995) while integrated *services* for persons with co-occurring disorders have superior results to parallel or sequential services (Jerrell & Ridgely, 1995). This indicates that integration is important at both the individual and system level. Additionally, service systems integration needs, but generally fails, to address the complex needs of service recipients, particularly for women with children (National Center for Service Integration, 1994). The gender-neutral framework of systems integration and the service system's relative inexperience in dealing with trauma places two requirements on systems integration strategies for this population. The strategies must develop networks of care as well as address the structural characteristics within these systems that create the potential for re-traumatization and ignore women's wholeness, complexity and self-described needs (Jennings, 1997; Veysey, 1997).

Rural Service Provision

Women residing in rural areas face additional challenges in receiving integrated and comprehensive services that are sensitive to the unique contexts of their lives. Barriers to service delivery include: physical isolation (Blank et al., 1996; Blank et al., 1995; Slaughter, 1990), transportation problems (Blank et al., 1996; Blank et al., 1995; Slaughter, 1990), conservatism and gender socialization (Slaughter, 1990), lack of privacy and fear of stigma (Wagenfeld et al., 1994), lack of culturally competent services (Chalifoux et al., 1996; Hill & Frasier, 1995), and weak linkages across systems (Chalifoux et al., 1996). Additionally, small town and rural gossip poses risks for women. Calls to the police and service seeking are likely to be known and may result in retaliation by husbands/partners, social exclusion and loss of child custody. Approaches that address some of these barriers include: (a) service outreach procedures (Blank et al., 1995); (b) informal resources as an adjunct to formal services (e.g., a Drop-in Center) (Bjorklund & Pippard, 1999); (c) in-home services (Blank et al., 1996); (d) alternative care providers (Windle, 1994); (e) culturally sensitive services (Chalifoux et al., 1996; Hill & Frasier, 1995); (f) innovative roles within the formal and informal support system for "consumers" (Bjorklund & Pippard, 1999); (g) inclusion of local communities and service recipients in policy and program development (Bjorklund & Pippard, 1999; Hill & Frasier, 1995); and (h) efforts to strengthen formal and informal linkages (Chalifoux et al., 1996).

What Helps Women Heal

Given that an individual's response to violence emerges from a complex interaction between the person, the event and the environment, posttraumatic responses and recovery vary widely. To be effective, interventions must be able to respond to the variety of personal, sociocultural, environmental, and interpersonal exigencies of individual women's lives (Harvey, 1996; Lebowitz et al., 1993). Women benefit from a treatment philosophy based on (a) competency building and empowerment; services and supports provided in safe, accessible and community-based locations (Alexander & Muenzenmaier, 1998); (b) mutual relationships built on trust, understanding and respect (Bassuk et al., 1998; Miller, 1990, 1994, 1996; Miller & Guidry, 2001; Prescott, 1998; Harris & Landis, 1997; Deegan, 1995; Unzicker, 1995); (c) the establishment and maintenance of safety (Hedges, 2000; Noble, 1999; Begley, 1998; Najavits et al., 1998; Talbott et al., 1998); and (d) trauma-specific treatment (Miller, 1990, 1994, 1996; Miller & Guidry, 2001; Harris & Landis, 1997; Harvey, 1991).

Women in this intervention present with a number of "clinical problems," including alcoholism, drug abuse and psychiatric illnesses. Women are also: (a) disenfranchised; (b) poor, un- or underemployed; (c) poorly educated with few marketable skills; and (d) socially isolated. The Project conducted focus groups in an effort to understand and respond to women's needs as they perceive them. The women revealed that they need jobs, friends, things to do, and therapists who treat them with respect. Women acknowledge the need for professional assistance to help them with their AOD and mental health problems, but place more value on other human needs and resources. The FCWVP incorporated knowledge from the women and the literature in designing the intervention.

TARGET POPULATION

Franklin County is largely rural with a total population of approximately 71,000 people spread across 30 towns and nearly 1,000 square miles. The racial, ethnic and cultural diversity of Franklin County is similar to poor, rural population pockets throughout New England. The county's ethnic/racial distribution is estimated to be 96% White/Non-Hispanic, 2% Hispanic, 1% African-American, and 1% Asian and Native American. Unemployment, poverty and violence rates rival those of urban centers (Armstrong & O'Brien, 1997). According to census data, the per capita personal income for Franklin County residents was $13,944, the lowest per capita income of all counties in Massachusetts (1990 US Census). Further, 31% of families with female heads of household and 67% of families with children under five years of age live below the nationally recognized poverty line (Official Income and Poverty Data for Franklin County, MA, Department of Public Health, 2000). Rates of assault, rape and child abuse are among the highest in the state (Armstrong & O'Brien, 1997). According to the Greenfield Recorder (1999), 39% of the calls to the Athol Police Department are related to domestic violence. Isolation is a profound problem, particularly in the outlying towns, which have spread out dwellings and limited transportation. The county has sparse health and behavioral health services. In fact, the federal government designated Franklin County as medically underserved based upon four criteria related to access to primary care: (a) percentage of the population below the poverty line; (b) percentage of the population over 65; (c) the infant mortality rate; and (d) number of primary care physicians.

Women participating in the intervention present a wide array of AOD and mental health problems. Many have experienced childhood sexual and physical abuse that persists into adulthood. Over 80% report emotional abuse and neglect, or physical or sexual abuse. Almost a third first experienced the abuse before the age of six. The women vary widely in age, parental status, sexual orientation, and location of residence. The mean age is 37, but ranges from 21 to 61. Seventy-nine percent have had children and 56% have lost legal custody of a child. Of those with children, 87% have children under the age of 18. A majority of the women live in their own apartment or house (57%). Women primarily identify as heterosexual (75%) and 47% are either married or have a significant other. The women have extensive involvement with formal treatment services; 86% were receiving services upon entering the study. Their psychiatric diagnoses vary from schizophrenia to borderline personality disorder; the primary substances of choice are alcohol and marijuana. Employment, education and income all reflect a group of women with limited means. Less than one-third of the women are employed and the mean yearly income of $12,556 is even less than the per capita income for the county as a whole. Twenty-seven percent do not have a high school diploma while 20% have a bachelor's degree or more.

PURPOSE AND GOALS

The primary purpose of the intervention design is to provide comprehensive, integrated, gender-specific, and trauma-informed AOD and mental health services within a resource poor community. Providing services and resources in a location with few formal treatment options presents a unique challenge. The systems integration strategy relies on maximizing the use of existing formal treatment services, while the individual-level services focus on mobilizing informal supports predominantly through the use of peer volunteers and natural community resources. Secondary goals include: (a) the specification of a rural, peer-driven services integration model; (b) the identification of specific challenges to treatment implicit in rural service delivery; and (c) information on how to develop working relationships across disciplines and philosophies. This information may be used to replicate this model in other communities to improve individual outcomes and reduce the use of expensive emergency or inpatient services.

DESCRIPTION OF THE INTERVENTION

Theoretical Underpinnings

The human potential movement provides the theoretical basis for the FCWVP. The intervention uses a blended theory that combines Maslow's (1970) hierarchy of needs, Herman's stages of recovery (1992), and the Stone Center's Relational Theory of women's recovery (Miller, 1976). The philosophy guiding Maslow's theory is that human beings have the capacity to reach their full potential and that unmet needs directly contribute to many problems that they encounter. Humans are primarily motivated by a push for physical and psychological survival and, when survival needs are met, by a push toward the actualization of inherent potentialities. Maslow identifies the hierarchy of needs as: (a) physical or basic needs, (b) safety, (c) love and belonging, (d) esteem, and (e) self-actualization. Previous levels' needs must be met before making significant progress in higher levels. This implies that individuals in recovery must have their basic needs met and be physically safe prior to making significant progress in their healing.

Herman (1992) suggests that abuse primarily results in disempowerment and disconnection from others; therefore, healing from trauma must focus on empowering the survivor and creating new connections with others.

Any therapeutic intervention that takes power away from the individual is counterproductive. In contrast, autonomy, which allows women to choose when and how they use treatment and other resources, promotes empowerment and recovery. Herman (1992) holds that recovery occurs in three stages: (a) safety, (b) remembrance and mourning, and (c) reconnection with ordinary life. These stages are a useful heuristic but should not be taken literally, nor are the stages necessarily linear (Herman, 1992). Safety includes naming the problem and creating emotional and physical safety. The second stage involves transforming the traumatic memory and mourning the losses. The third stage, reconnection, includes learning to fight, reconciling with oneself, reconnecting with others, finding a survivor mission, and resolving the trauma.

Relational Theory (Miller, 1976) provides the final component for the Project model. Growing evidence supports the hypothesis that women differ significantly from men physiologically, developmentally, experientially, and socially. These differences exemplify the need for gender-specific approaches to healing. Relational Theory adopts a gender-specific approach and states that empowering relationships between women and those around them is the primary mechanism by which women heal (Miller, 1976).

Blending the three theories together with experiential knowledge derived from the Project led to the development of the following heuristic model (see Figure 1). The model begins with addressing women's basic needs, such as food, shelter and clothing, and establishing physical safety prior to any therapeutic or support intervention then moves onto changing women's relationships, roles and sense of self. Empowering relationships (i.e., relationships that support the value and humanity of the individual while setting appropriate boundaries between individuals) serve as the linchpin of recovery and wellness. Relationships allow women to explore new roles and skills, both vocational and relational. More important than the simple accumulation of skills is the assumption of valued roles (i.e., roles that the community at large value, such as skilled daycare worker, computer operator, therapy group leader). Skill development and the assumption of valued roles help build self-esteem and self-efficacy. Experiences in relationships and in developing new skills and roles change the way women view themselves and their own histories. For example, women may redefine their primary identity from alcoholic to survivor to peer resource advocate.

At this point, women begin to see their traumatic experiences less as wounds and more as assets. The concept of self-actualization embodies this and is comprised of three distinct constructs: (a) recontextualization

FIGURE 1. Heuristic Model of Woman-Centered Growth Potential

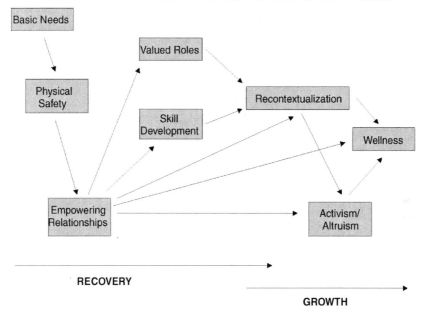

(i.e., the ability of individuals to reframe their experiences and redefine themselves) (Way, 1962), (b) activism/altruism (i.e., the ability to reach beyond oneself in the service of causes or individuals) (Frankl, 1978), and (c) wellness (Higgins, 1994). The ability to (a) give and receive love and acceptance in relationship, (b) change their perceptions of self in the world (i.e., come to love and value themselves) and (c) provide support for causes and/or individuals define wellness.

While this woman-centered human potential model best describes the philosophy of the Project, the process of recovery from AOD addiction and distressing mental health symptoms requires further clarification. This model assumes a relationship between trauma (especially childhood occurrence) and adult AOD use, psychiatric disorders, and adaptive strategies that are often interpreted as symptoms of psychiatric disorders. Trauma is primary while psychiatric disorders and alcohol and other drug problems are secondary responses. This has clear implications for therapeutic interventions in an integrated trauma-informed system: specifically, trauma must be addressed directly while emotional distress and adaptive strategies, such as addiction, also require attention even if they are not the primary focus. Women may access resources to address specific problems (e.g., alcoholism, emotional distress, mental health concerns, self-esteem, trauma). However, the recovery process does not theoretically require women to focus on deficits. In fact, this model predicts a decrease in AOD use and mental health symptoms as women engage in supportive relationships, skills building, meaningful work, and valued roles.

The Service Model

The three Drop-in Centers serve as the focal points of the individual level intervention. Following the logic of the heuristic model, FCWVP services and supports incorporate four core elements: (a) safe space, (b) trauma groups, (c) peer resource advocacy, and (d) opportunities for valued roles. Each Drop-in Center provides all four core elements of the intervention that are offered in sequence: (a) physically safe space in the drop-in centers establishes a sense of safety; (b) the trauma group (i.e., ATRIUM model) provides women with connections to others, empowering relationships, tools to recontextualize earlier experiences, and methods of self-care; (c) peer resource advocates help women meet self-identified needs and goals, establish links to the community, and identify opportunities for skill development; and (d) opportunities for valued roles offer a sense of worth and self-efficacy as well as concrete employment transferable skills.

Safe Space and Other Services, Supports, and Resources. The three Drop-in Centers provide physically safe, peer-run, women-only space. None of the Centers have time limits on use of services and resources. The Centers offer other resources in addition to the core services. The Survivor's Project at the Long Street House is located on a public transportation line in Greenfield, the largest and most centrally located community in the county. The Center offers AA meetings, an art room, quiet room, resource library, free childcare and children's play room, a large garden, free clothing exchange, computer and Internet access, a healthy midday meal, expressive and creative groups (e.g., writing, yoga, theater), training and workshops, and a comfortable space to relax. The Center is open about 50 hours/week (M-F 9-5 and some evenings). CSR-identified women comprise 50% of the staff and 75% of the volunteers who assist in running the Center.

Day Break Drop-in Center in Orange/Athol provides drop-in space in the northeast portion of Franklin County with a quiet room, a resource room, childcare and children's activities, laundry facilities, free clothing and furniture exchange, and rooms for temporary shelter. The Center is open about 50 hours/week (M-F 9-5 and some evenings). Staffing consists of a full-time Program Coordinator, volunteers and support from staff at the Orange Family Inn next door. The third center, the Catholic Family Services Drop-in Center, is in Montague. There women may connect and access resources, including computers and educational resources, childcare and children's programs, mothering support activities, and a free clothing exchange room. The Center is open roughly 20 hours/week during evenings and weekends. Staffing consists of one half-time Program Coordinator, with support from on-site volunteers.

The ATRIUM Model. The Addictions and Trauma Recovery Integration Model (ATRIUM) is a manualized, trauma recovery program. It is an effective bio-psychosocial group intervention that responds to the complex treatment needs of trauma survivors. Groups provide trauma survivors with safety and human connections that help participants learn valuable coping skills and gain a sense of hopefulness (Najavits et al., 1998; Chard et al., 1997; Stein & Eisen, 1996). ATRIUM cultivates a more holistic treatment paradigm and understanding of trauma by actively identifying and exploring the mind/body interface in relation to trauma (Miller & Guidry, 2001). The focus on trauma and addictions provides an opportunity for women to recontextualize their experiences and adaptive strategies. Each group has two facilitators, one of whom is a trauma survivor/CSR. A licensed psychologist trains and supervises the facilitators. Each group meets for one session (1.5 hours) per week for 12 weeks. ATRIUM has been found to decrease depression, externalized forms of self-soothing, such as self-harm, suicidality and aggression; it also reduces intrusive symptoms associated with PTSD (Miller & Guidry, 2001).

Peer Resource Advocates. Peer Resource Advocates (PRAs) combine strength-based case management with an empowerment model. The "consumer-driven" strengths model focuses on improving each woman's quality of life by identifying and enriching her individual strengths, and accessing resources needed for community integration (Stanard, 1999). PRAs are women with similar AOD, trauma and mental health experiences who are further along in their healing and interested in reaching out to other women. This model is inherently empowering for both women in the partnership: the advocates represent a source of hope, possibility and capacity for women coming into the project; at the same time, the PRAs experience themselves as competent and contributing to someone else's well-being. The approach is highly individualized, focusing on concrete supports and specific skill-building.

PRAs help women articulate their own strengths, needs and goals, and then access resources in the community that foster healing and growth. Recognizing the unique barriers faced by poor, rural women, PRAs are mobile. They can meet with women in their homes, at the Drop-in Centers or other locations. Staffing consists of one full-time Volunteer Coordinator, based at the Survivor's Project, who handles recruitment, training, supervision, and support of the 15-20 trained volunteer PRAs. In addition, staff at the other two Centers provides support and coordination for PRAs at these sites. PRAs work with individual women for 1-3 hours/week over a period of 16 weeks and, at a minimum, help them develop an individual Wellness Recovery Action Plan (WRAP).

Valued Social Roles. The Project offers opportunities to gain skills and assume new roles. Women may volunteer or work as paid staff for the Project (e.g., field researchers, PRAs, group co-facilitators, committee members). Women may also volunteer to run the Drop-in Centers (e.g., childcare workers, gardeners, cooks, and greeters). These opportunities for valued social roles benefit both the women served by the Project and the Project itself. Women experience themselves and are seen by others as worthy and capable of making valuable contributions. The Volunteer PRA Coordinator, Program Coordinator, CSR Coordinator, Principal Investigator, Co-Principal Investigator, and ATRIUM and Ethnography Supervisor all support the women in their roles. This element of the intervention does not have specific staffing requirements. The hours per week and duration of involvement depend on each woman.

Clinical/Individual Level Services Integration Strategies

Services integration at the individual level is peer-delivered and accomplished through (a) the ATRIUM groups (an integrated trauma/mental health and addiction model); (b) co-location of peer-run or -supported trauma services (e.g., ATRIUM groups and other trauma-specific supports), AOD services (e.g., AA meetings), and mental health services (e.g., Wellness Recovery Action Plan Group, groups addressing self-esteem, etc.) at the Drop-in Centers; and (c) PRAs who help women identify and access mental health, AOD, trauma and other services that interest them. All three Centers use these integrated strategies.

Organizational/Program Level Services Integration Strategies

The FCWVP organizational/program level services integration utilizes a number of strategies. They include the "Trauma Liaison" position, various county level policy and practice committees, and cross-training. The Trauma Liaison, who is funded by the FCWVP and housed at the Franklin Medical Center (FMC), acts as a boundary span-ner chairing the Integration and Policy Committees. The Liaison: (a) fosters collaboration and alliances among county agencies; (b) over-sees joint development of memoranda of understanding (MOUs), poli-cies and procedures; (c) facilitates cross-system communication and knowledge exchange; (d) participates in case conferences, providing a comprehensive trauma perspective; and (e) acts as consultant on trauma issues for women in FMC emergency room, AOD and mental health treatment services.

Policy and practice committees include the Integration Committee and the Policy Committee. The FCWVP Integration Committee meets bi-monthly and focuses on improving treatment practices among pro-viders. The Committee: (a) works to improve mental health and AOD services; (b) develops practices that foster a comprehensive, coordi-nated, CSR-involved array of trauma-informed services for women, in-cluding outreach and engagement, screening and assessment, treatment activities, parenting support and education, resource coordination and advocacy, trauma-specific services, crisis intervention, and peer-run ser-vices; (c) promotes collaborative relationships, knowledge exchange, and effective communication across partner organizations; (d) develops uni-versal screening criteria; and (e) develops a referral mechanism to facili-tate access to all core services regardless of a woman's initial point of entry. The FCWVP Policy Committee also meets bi-monthly to develop policies that support a comprehensive, integrated, and trauma-sensitive community of care for women that is informed by a CSR perspective. The Policy Committee supports the development of agency policies, policy consistency across agencies, formal working agreements among "close-in" partner agencies and training. These elements provide envi-ronmental support for integrated and trauma-informed clinical practice and programs.

Community Development

Communities, like individuals, can be stressed. As noted above, Franklin County is an extremely impoverished and isolated area. While no community member admits to contributing to violence, the culture supports violence and the silence surrounding it. Like the women in the Project, community recovery requires a process of naming and reclaim-ing, supported by resources. No anti-violence project can be successful for long if the community in which it is imbedded embraces the values of violence. The FCWVP utilized two strategies to increase community awareness of trauma issues and to support community development: (a) a broad-based media and training focus and (b) the creation of employment opportunities.

The FCWVP sought out media opportunities to discuss trauma in general and Project activities in specific. Several television public service announcements, TV news reports and newspaper articles were presented during this time. The Project supported, and made open to all community members, extensive cross-system training opportunities on topics such as the intersection of trauma, mental health and AOD, unlearning the "client" role, hearing voices, self-injury, conflict resolution, and communication.

Internships and volunteer positions were integral to developing skills transferable to employment opportunities. Equally important was the use of Project funds to support Community Initiative Grants. Local individuals and groups received these small grants to subsidize resources, such as acupuncture, massage, reiki treatments and practitioner training. The Community Initiative Grants did not focus on any particular area, but were designed to be responsive to the self-identified needs of the community.

Finally, to enhance knowledge and foster a better understanding of trauma in the community at large, the FCWVP established a Coordinating Council. This Council brings together representatives from a broad array of community agencies, such as service providers, schools and educators, social services and housing representatives, church leaders, and emergency response staff (i.e., police and emergency medical) on a quarterly basis. Its goals are to foster awareness of violence and its consequences, create a forum for networking and discussion around trauma-related issues, and develop trauma-informed community resources.

CENTRAL ROLE OF CONSUMER/SURVIVOR/ RECOVERING (CSR) WOMEN

Since CSR women and their allies conceptualized, developed, implemented and evaluated the entire project, the concept of "CSR Integration" as generally understood does not capture the approach and philosophy of the FCWVP. We see the involvement of CSR women (both professionals and non-professional local women) as a strategy for better understanding and addressing the impact of trauma on women's lives and the lives of their children, rather than as an end in and of itself.

CSR women lead, advise, administer and evaluate the work of this project. The Principal Investigator and much of the senior staff (seven out of 11) making up the Executive Committee (the major decision-making body) identify as CSRs. Local CSR women are members of the FCWVP Coordinating Council and Integration and Policy Committees; women participate through community meetings in decision making for activities and programming at the Survivor's Project. The Women's Advisory Committee, which is made up of paid CSR women, meets between two and four times a month to discuss and provide input on Project and research activities. A CSR Coordinator acts as a liaison between local women involved with the Project and the activities of the National Steering Committee. CSR volunteers do a majority of the work associated with running the Drop-in Centers, including acting as ATRIUM and other group leaders (e.g., yoga, writing), PRAs, childcare workers, cooks, and office staff. Finally, the research team includes numerous CSRs. Both the Co-Principal Investigator and ATRIUM and Ethnography Supervisor are women who identify as CSRs. Three local CSR-identified women (without research skills or experience) joined the research team at the outset as research interns in order to both influence the planning and implementation of the local and multi-site evaluation, as well as to develop useful, transferable research skills. All three interns were subsequently offered positions as paid field researchers. CSR-identified women also worked as interviewers for the outcome study.

Women also serve on an ad-hoc basis on hiring committees for Project positions (e.g., Trauma Liaison). Finally, through focus groups (most recently as part of an asset-based community assessment), local CSR women have identified strengths and gaps in the service system and community with respect to availability, accessibility and trauma sensitivity of supports and resources for women and their children. CSR women (both professional and non-professional) provided many unique perspectives throughout the development of the local evaluation and cross-site studies. Their input and involvement have been integral and invaluable to the research and to the local research participants. The evolution of the project has been not only profoundly influenced, but also genuinely driven, by CSR-identified women.

LESSONS LEARNED

Lessons learned from the implementation process underscore the notion that community change is the key to individual recovery. Changing the social environment in which women with histories of violence live creates safety not only for those women, but also for other citizens. A community that values non-violence will challenge institutional practices that re-traumatize persons in its care. This supports women's individual efforts to overcome the effects of violence.

Paradigm Development

The first two years of the FCWVP focused on developing a shared division, which was arguably the most difficult aspect of the Project. Members of the Executive Committee came from a variety of backgrounds and training; they argued and disagreed until reaching a consensus on key issues: (a) the role of trauma in the causal sequence of AOD and mental health problems, (b) primary healing trajectories, (c) key points of intervention, and (d) resources necessary to fill in the gaps. This ongoing discussion was essential. The time spent in hammering out principles and goals invested the lead agencies and local women in the activities of the Project. In some cases, this was the first time treatment and advocacy agencies met with persons in their care. The resulting Project is grounded in the real life experiences of local women and affects all treatment services in Franklin County.

Mobilizing Local Resources

While this project focuses on integrating AOD and mental health treatment, the necessities of rural life require mobilization of other local resources. Treatment services are sparse and located only in the largest community (with minimal support in one other community). This means that the vast majority of women cannot easily access services. First responders, such as EMTs and police, are the *de facto* emergency behavioral health providers. Many other organizations also provide "treatment" for women. These include: ministers, imams and rabbis; peer groups, such as AA; libraries through public service meetings and discussions; school staff; homeless/battered women shelters; and social services. Unavailability and poor access to the formal treatment system in resource poor communities necessitates the mobilization of these natural support systems to provide a safety net. The close-knit nature of rural communities facilitates this type of broad-based collaboration since community members know each other. Mobilizing natural resources creates 24-hour, seven day a week support for isolated women. In addition, these supports tend to be less intrusive and stigmatizing than formal treatment services.

Bridging the Gaps

The AOD, mental health and domestic violence paradigms differ significantly in most clinical domains, including causation, treatment, and prognosis. Past research demonstrates that parallel or sequential treatment is less effective than integrated treatment. In fact, treating one disorder or issue without considering the effects of other intersecting issues can be detrimental or even injurious. Creating clinical integration requires that all participating clinicians broaden their professional paradigms. In practice, this requires cross-training, a mechanism for cross-agency discussion and collaboration, shared assessment and treatment planning, and trauma-specific troubleshooting and technical assistance. The Trauma Liaison has been invaluable in creating these resources.

The Value of Peer-Led Services

Women need to trust and feel comfortable in a therapeutic environment. A non-judgmental attitude that validates each woman's experiences and feelings is essential. For many women this means talking to others who have had similar experiences and can empathize with her; women value these interactions. Peer supports, whether in groups or other settings, offer several benefits. The interactions demonstrate to women that they are not alone and that others have experienced similar traumatic events. Just as women find it helpful when someone listens to them, listening to others talk about their experiences aids in healing. Seeing others who are not as far along in their recovery helps women see the progress they have made. Conversely, seeing what others have accomplished demonstrates the potential to heal and have a life that is not dictated by alcohol, drugs, trauma, or mental health issues. Taken one step further, role modeling provides an opportunity to help others as well as an incentive to keep moving forward so as to not set a poor example. Additionally, helping others can transform the traumatic experience into something that benefits others.

Challenges and Rewards of CSR Training

CSR-identified women struggle day-to-day with long-standing issues and have enormous strengths learned as survivors. They also face significant difficulties resulting from persistent challenges to their self-esteem. The CSRs in this project, from trained professionals to volunteers and interns, all face the residual effects of the experienced trauma, particularly the emotionality of the topic area itself. The women are extremely committed to this issue and Project success; they put heart and soul into their work. On the other hand, failure looms larger–out of perspective to the actual events.

Training to increase individual skills is the easy part. Providing emotional support and day-to-day guidance to assure each woman that she is doing well is both time consuming and exhausting. In the end both CSRs and the Project benefit. The CSRs have new skills, confidence in their abilities, an understanding of the research and practical issues that is informed by their own experience, and have transformed the meaning of their trauma from injury to asset. The Project, both program and research, has benefited from their insight and guidance.

CONCLUSION

The FCWVP is an ongoing set of interventions and community development strategies for women with co-occurring disorders and histories of violence. The effectiveness of the ATRIUM model; accompanying services, supports and resources; and the services and systems integration strategies undertaken in this project have yet to be determined. However, integrated, multidisciplinary, trauma-informed/specific services that are sensitive to women's individual contexts and needs are sorely lacking and findings from this study should prove instrumental in designing comprehensive, integrated services for this group of women. The implementation process has informed the field on the challenges and benefits of rural services integration. The heavy focus on peer support and CSR involvement in the development and implementation of this model is unique and provides an opportunity to assess the impact of a peer-driven model on healing and recovery. The hope is that the principles applied here can be applied elsewhere when done with careful consideration for the resources, level of systems and services integration, gender and cultural sensitivity, and degree of trauma awareness in the community.

REFERENCES

Alexander M.J., & Muenzenmaier, K. (1998). Trauma, addiction and recovery: Addressing public health epidemics among women with severe mental illness. In B.L. Levin, A. Blanch, and A. Jennings (Eds.), *Women's Mental Health Services: A Public Health Perspective* (pp. 215-39). Thousand Oaks, CA: Sage Publications.

Begley, E.A. (1998). A narrative study of inpatient experiences of female child sexual abuse survivors. Dissertation Abstracts International: The Sciences and Engineering. 58(10-B): 5635.

Bevett-Mills, J. (2000). Quote from the following article by Barton, J.: Violence against women: SAMHSA's response. *SAMHSA News, 8*(4), 5-8.

Bjorklund, R.W. & Pippard, J.L. (1999). The mental health consumer movement: Implications for rural practice. *Community Mental Health Journal, 35*(4), 347-359.

Blanch, A.K. & Levin, B.L. (1998). Organization and services delivery. In B.L. Levin, and A.K. Blanch (Eds.), *Women's Mental Health Services: A Public Health Perspective* (pp. 5-18). Thousand Oaks, CA: Sage Publications.

Blanch, A.K., Nicholson, J., & Purcell, J. (1994). Parents with severe mental illness and their children: The need for human services integration. *Journal of Mental Health Administration, 21*(4), 388-396.

Blank, M.B., Jodl, K.M., & McCall, B.R. (1996). Psychosocial rehabilitation program characteristics in urban and rural areas. *Psychiatric Rehabilitation Journal, 20*, 3-10.

Blank, M.B., Fox, J.C., Hargrove, D.S., & Turner, J.T. (1995). Critical issues in reforming rural mental health service delivery. *Community Mental Health Journal, 31*(6), 511-524.

Carlson, E.B, Furby, L., Armstrong, J., & Shlaes, J. (1997). A conceptual framework for the long-term psychological effects of traumatic childhood abuse. *Child Maltreatment: Journal of the American Professional Society on the Abuse of Children, 2*(3), 272-295.

Carmen, E.H., Crane, B., Dunnicliff, M., Holochuck, S., Prescott, L., Rieker, P.P., Stefan, S., & Stromberg, N. (1996). *Massachusetts Department of Mental Health Task Force on the Restraint and Seclusion of Persons Who Have Been Physically or Sexually Abused: Report and Recommendations.* Boston, MA: Department of Mental Health.

Chalifoux, Z., Neese, J.B., Buckwalter, K.C., Litwak, E. et al. (1996). Mental health services for rural elderly: Innovative service strategies. *Community Mental Health Journal, 32*(5), 463-480.

Chard, K.M., Weaver, T.L. & Resick, P.A. (1997). Adapting cognitive processing therapy for child sexual abuse survivors. *Cognitive and Behavioral Practice, 4*(1), 31-52.

Commonwealth Fund. (1997). *Facts on Abuse and Violence: The Commonwealth Fund Survey of the Health of Adolescent Girls.* New York: Louis Harris and Associates, Inc.

Deegan, P.E. (1995). Recovery as a journey of the heart. Paper presented at the Conference for Recovery from Psychiatric Disability, Boston, May 10, 1995.

Frankl, V.E. (1978). *The Unheard Cry for Meaning: Psychotherapy and Humanism.* New York, NY: Simon and Schuster.

Harris, M. & Landis, C.L. (Eds.) (1997). *Sexual Abuse in the Lives of Women Diagnosed with Serious Mental Illness.* Netherlands: Harwood Academic Publishers.

Harris, M. & The Community Connections Trauma Work Group. (1998). *Trauma Recovery and Empowerment: A Clinician's Guide To Working with Women in Groups.* New York: Free Press.

Harris, M. (1994). Modifications in service delivery and clinical treatment for women diagnosed with severe mental illness who are also the survivors of trauma. Special

Issue: Women's mental health services. *Journal of Mental Health Administration,* *21*(4), 397-406.

Harvey, M. (1996). An ecological view of psychological trauma and trauma recovery. *Journal of Traumatic Stress, 9,* 3-23.

Hedges, L.E. (2000). *Terrifying Transferences: Aftershocks of Childhood Trauma.* Northvale, New Jersey: Jason Aronson, Inc.

Herman, J.L. (1992). *Trauma and Recovery: The Aftermath of Violence–From Domestic Abuse to Political Terror.* New York: Basic Books.

Higgins, G.O. (1994). *Resilient Adults: Overcoming a Cruel Past.* San Francisco, CA: Jossey-Bass.

Hill, C.E. & Fraser, G.J. (1995). Local knowledge and rural mental health reform. *Community Mental Health Journal, 31*(6), 553-568.

Jennings, A. (1997). On being invisible in the mental health system. In M. Harris & C. Landis (Eds.), *Sexual Abuse in the Lives of Women Diagnosed with Serious Mental Illness* (pp. 162-180). Netherlands: Harwood Academic Publishers.

Jerrell, J.M. & Ridgely, M.S. (1995). Comparative effectiveness of three approaches to serving people with severe mental illness and substance abuse disorders. *Journal of Nervous and Mental Disease, 183*(9): 566-576.

Lebowitz, L., Harvey, M.R., & Herman, J.L. (1993). A stage-by-dimension model of recovery from sexual trauma. *Journal of Interpersonal Violence, 8*(3), 378-391.

Levin, B.L. & Blanch, A.K. (Eds.) (1998). *Women's Mental Health Services: A Public Health Perspective.* Thousand Oaks, CA: Sage Publications.

Maslow, A.H. 1970. *Motivation and Personality* (2nd ed.). New York: Harper and Row.

Miller, A. (1990). *Banished Knowledge: Facing Childhood Injuries.* New York: Doubleday.

Miller, D. (1994). *Women Who Hurt Themselves.* New York: Basicbooks.

Miller, D. (1996). Challenging self-harm through transformation of the trauma story. *Sexual Addiction and Compulsivity, 3*(3), 213-227.

Miller, D. & Guidry, L. (2001). *Addictions and Trauma Recovery: Healing the Body, Mind and Spirit.* New York: W.W. Norton.

Miller, J.B. (1976). *Toward a New Psychology of Women.* Boston: Beacon Press.

Morrissey, J.P., Johnsen, M.C., & Calloway, M.O. (1993). "Systems analysis of children's mental health service networks." Presented at the Annual Meeting of the American Public Health Association, San Francisco, CA.

Najavits, L.M., Weiss, R.D., Shaw, S.R., & Muenz, L.R. (1998). "Seeking safety": Outcome of a new cognitive-behavioral psychotherapy for women with posttraumatic stress disorder and substance dependence. *Journal of Traumatic Stress, 11*(3), 437-456.

National Center for Service Integration. (1994). "Providing Comprehensive Integrated Services for Children and Families: Why Is It So Hard?" *NCSI News,* Winter: 1-3.

Noble, S.C. (1999). Nondiscursive communication in the psychotherapeutic encounter: An analysis of practitioners' experiences with clients exhibiting symptoms of trauma. *Dissertation Abstracts International: The Sciences and Engineering.* 59(8-B): 4011.

Oyserman, D., Mowbray, C.T., & Zemencuk, J.K. (1994). Resources and supports for mothers with severe mental illness. *Health and Social Work, 19*(2), 132-141.

Slaughter, C. (1990). "Starting a Rural Project for Women." *NCADV Voice*, Winter, 1-2, 6.

Stanard, R.P. (1999). The effect of training in a strengths model of case management on client outcomes in a community mental health center. *Community Mental Health Journal, 35*(2), 169-179.

Stein, E.J. & Eisen, B. (1996). Helping trauma survivors cope: Effects of immediate brief co-therapy and crisis intervention. *Crisis Intervention and Time-Limited Treatment, 3*(2), 113-127.

Talbott, J.A. (1995). Evaluation the Johnson Foundation program on chronic mental illness: An interview with Howard Goldman. *Psychiatric Services, 45*(5), 501-503.

Unzicker, R. (1995). From the inside. In J. Grobe (Ed.), *Beyond Bedlam: Contemporary Psychiatric Survivors Speak Out* (pp. 13-18). Chicago: Third Side Press.

Veysey, B.M. (1997). Specific needs of women diagnosed with mental illness in U.S. jails. In B.L. Levin, and A.K. Blanch (Eds.), *Women's Mental Health Services: A Public Health Perspective* (pp. 368-89). Thousand Oaks, CA: Sage Publications.

Wagenfeld, M.O., Murray, J.D., Mohatt, D.F., & DeBruyn, J.C. (1994) *Mental Health and Rural America: 1980-1993*. Washington, DC: Public Health Service.

Way, L. (1962). *Adler's Place in Psychology*. New York: Collier Books.

Windle, C. (1994). Social values and services research: The case of rural services. *Administration and Policy in Mental Health, 22*(2), 181-188.

Creating Alcohol and Other Drug, Trauma, and Mental Health Services for Women in Rural Florida: The Triad Women's Project

Colleen Clark, PhD
Julienne Giard, PhD
Margo Fleisher-Bond, MA
Sharon Slavin
Marion Becker, PhD
Arthur Cox, DSW, LCSW

SUMMARY. Located in central Florida, the Triad Women's Project is a comprehensive system of care developed to respond to the needs of women and children living in a three-county semi-rural area. The women have histories of abuse or violence, co-occurring alcoholism and other drug (AOD) and mental health disorders, and have been high utililizers

Colleen Clark and Julienne Giard are affiliated with the University of South Florida, Florida Mental Health Institute. Margo Fleisher-Bond and Sharon Slavin are affiliated with the Triad Women's Project. Marion Becker is affiliated with the University of South Florida, Florida Mental Health Institute. Arthur Cox is affiliated with the Florida Center for Addictions and Dual Disorders.

The authors wish to acknowledge Tri-County Human Services, Inc. and the Behavioral Health Division at Winter Haven Hospital, the two lead agencies that implemented the Triad Services, for their work on and commitment to the Triad Women's Project.

[Haworth co-indexing entry note]: "Creating Alcohol and Other Drug, Trauma, and Mental Health Services for Women in Rural Florida: The Triad Women's Project." Clark, Colleen et al. Co-published simultaneously in *Alcoholism Treatment Quarterly* (The Haworth Press, Inc.) Vol. 22, No. 3/4, 2004, pp. 41-61; and: *Responding to Physical and Sexual Abuse in Women with Alcohol and Other Drug and Mental Disorders: Program Building* (ed: Bonita M. Veysey, and Colleen Clark) The Haworth Press, Inc., 2004, pp. 41-61. Single or multiple copies of this article are available for a fee from The Haworth Document Delivery Service [1-800-HAWORTH, 9:00 a.m. - 5:00 p.m. (EST). E-mail address: docdelivery@haworthpress.com].

of behavioral healthcare services. This paper will describe the efforts of collaborating providers, the women themselves, services researchers, and concerned community members to develop services to assist these women in their AOD recovery, their healing from abuse, and their empowerment in dealing with mental illnesses. Practical information on establishing consensus, dealing with barriers and filling service gaps will be presented. *[Article copies available for a fee from The Haworth Document Delivery Service: 1-800-HAWORTH. E-mail address: <docdelivery@haworthpress. com> Website: <http://www.HaworthPress.com> © 2004 by The Haworth Press, Inc. All rights reserved.]*

KEYWORDS. Alcoholism, drug abuse, women, physical abuse, sexual abuse, rural

STATEMENT OF THE PROBLEM

Women with co-occurring alcoholism and other drug problems (AOD) and mental health problems and histories of abuse have diverse problems in many areas of their lives. At the individual level, they struggle with the effects of the violence they have experienced, dependence or abuse of alcohol and other drugs, and a range of mental and emotional problems. They are incarcerated at times and struggle with the responsibilities of parenting, sometimes losing custody of their children, either permanently or temporarily. At the systems level, the women sometimes are unable to get services they need, find it difficult to stay in AOD programs, or relapse because of emotional problems or inability to resolve trauma-related issues, and often are unable to get help or medication for problems, such as depression. Mental health programs often lack attention to AOD issues and sometimes deny services to people who are struggling with AOD problems. Overriding many of these problems, women worry about surviving in the world outside their treatment programs. This includes finding a safe, affordable place to live, satisfying work and transportation, and for those that have children, making a good home for their children.

People with co-occurring disorders need integrated care (Carey, 1996), but services are often fragmented. A review of Florida's Alcohol, Drug, and Mental Health (ADM) system by the State's Office of Program Policy Analysis and Government Accountability (1999) concluded that lack of coordination between service providers was the system's biggest deficiency. There are two fairly distinct funding streams for AOD and mental health programs making access to appropriate care for this target population difficult regardless of which gateway they enter treatment, not unlike many other services systems (Ridgely, Goldman, & Willenbring, 1990). The Robert Wood Johnson Fort Bragg study reminds us that system change must be addressed at both the system and service levels (Ridgely, Lambert, Goodman, Chichester, & Ralph, 1998). Further, the burden of treatment consistency and continuity needs to be placed with staff and not consumers (Zweben, 1996).

The cost of few or inappropriate services to this vulnerable population is staggering. Inadequate and inappropriate services reduces the quality of life of these women and their children and increases the cost to many other systems in our society, including criminal justice, welfare, healthcare, juvenile justice, and child welfare. For example, in 1997, illicit AOD increased Florida's hospitals' costs by $304 million. More than $250 million of these increased costs covered hospitalizations for diseases and other health disorders caused or exacerbated by AOD (State of Florida Agency for Healthcare Administration, 1999).

TARGET POPULATION

Women served by the Triad Women's Project live and receive services in a three-county (i.e., Polk, Highlands, and Hardee) semi-rural area in Florida designated District 14 by the state Department of Children and Families. The project implemented a number of strategies during the developmental phase to identify and describe the women to be served (see Table 1). Ten women were interviewed extensively to better understand their lives, their histories and current situations, and their attempts to receive services. One hundred thirty-one women participated in earlier versions of the interventions and were administered demographic and other surveys to assess their response to these interventions. Sixty-nine women were involved in focus groups in different settings including treatment settings, jails, domestic violence shelters and consumer drop-in centers. Information was also gathered from jail statistics, the results of biopsychosocial interviews at dependency court, chart reviews at one inpatient setting, and from key informants at service agencies in the district.

The women are, on average, in their mid-thirties. Almost all of the women (78-100%) have had multiple treatment episodes and are therefore "high end users." They describe many episodes of short-term, usually unsuccessful stays in detox units, psychiatric crisis stabilization

TABLE 1. Triad Target Population Descriptors from Various Sources

	Pilot Studies	Case History	Focus Groups	Jails	Dependency Court	Chart Review	Key Informant
Number of Women	131	10	69	288	41	100	12,296
Average Age	33.5	35.4		38		35.7	
Abuse History: Any	85%	90%	100%		56%	72%	62%
In childhood	63.7%		28%			51%	
Any sexual abuse	77%					48%	
Diagnoses: Average number	3.09					2.98	
Both MH and SA diagnoses	99%				76%	100%	36%
PTSD	30%					14%	
Treatment History: High end user	86%		78%			100%	
Children: % of women w/ children	79.4%	100%	91%		100%	76%	75%
# of dependent children	265					150	
Average # of children	2.55					1.97	
Race/Ethnicity: Black	25%	20%	32%	34%		21%	
White	63%	60%	65%	67%		66%	
Hispanic	7%	20%	3%			11%	
Other	5%					2%	
Marital Status: Married	15%	50%					
Separated	23%	20%					
Divorced	27%	10%					
Widowed	3%						
Never married	32%	20%					
Education: Less than H.S. grad	40.5%	50%					
High school grad or more	58.0%	50%					
Court-Ordered to Treatment	32.8%				100%		

units, and emergency rooms. The great majority of women in all of the settings report being victims of violence at some time in their lives (56-100%). Of those who participated in our pilot studies, 58% reported both physical and sexual abuse, 64% were abused as children, and 66% report that their abusers were family members.

Table 1 clearly illustrates the prevalence of co-occurring disorders, and the average number of diagnoses is three. In the pilot studies, about 30% of the women had been diagnosed with PTSD. Of those who have children (about 75%), the average number of diagnoses is two. A more detailed picture of the status of these women's children emerges in our review of 100 charts of women in treatment for co-occurring disorders. About 18% of the women had lost custody of their children, and the children were either in foster care, adopted out, or with family members. More frequently, about 30% of the time, their children were in the temporary custody of others, usually extended family, the children's father or a friend. Remarkably, in the focus groups and case history interviews, all of the women expressed concerns about problems their children were experiencing, most frequently behavioral problems followed closely by AOD.

The women in this three county area are primarily Caucasian (see Table 1). The predominant racial minority is African American women (14%). Hispanic women comprise the second largest ethnic minority group. Women who identify themselves as having Hispanic ethnic origins have many different cultural backgrounds, including Mexican, Cuban, Puerto Rican, other Central American, and other Caribbean. Hardee is the smallest of the counties; 28.4% of the people in this country are of Hispanic ethnicity and there is a significant Haitian population.

Special Ethnic Studies

To better understand the unique ethnic needs of Haitian women and their families, we commissioned an ethnographic study by a Creole speaking anthropologist. The study was conducted over a 3-month period in 1999. Through observations and interviews, her general findings were that there was a great deal of denial in the community around AOD, that the women's lives were impacted by the AOD of the men in their lives and the resulting violence, they had difficulties using domestic violence shelters, and that issues around abuse and violence were embedded in a culture of patriarchal domination. At the same time, help and support for all these issues was described as coming from families and the Haitian community itself.

While Hispanic women make up the largest ethnic minority in District 14, we found so few Hispanic women in the traditional behavioral healthcare agencies that Spanish speaking interviewers went to the jails to learn more about their lives. These women were incarcerated for drug-related charges or for probation violations. They reported long histories of violence and abuse, as children and adults. Most began using drugs as a result of relationships with drug users. Like Triad women of all ethnicities, a primary concern was their children. They reported feeling isolated from traditional cultural supports due to ostracization or feelings of shame about their drug abuse and domestic violence.

To better understand the special needs and circumstances of African American women, it is important to understand the socioeconomic environment of central Florida and Florida in general.The mean household income for a white home is $38,000, for those with Hispanic origins it is $33,000, but for black homes it is only $24,000. Further evidence of the systemic racism in this area is a comparison of incarceration rates. In these three counties, African Americans make up 14% of the general population, but 46% of incarcerated offenders (Bureau of Economic and Business Research, 1999). Data from the pilot interventions were examined and a few issues stand out. Black and Hispanic women were more likely to have children. Hispanic women in treatment tended to be older, more likely to be married, and much more likely to be court-ordered to treatment. Black women reported lower rates of sexual abuse, while Hispanic women were less likely to have experienced their abuse by a family member. There were no differences in terms of number of diagnoses, but black women were much more likely to be diagnosed with drug dependence, especially cocaine dependence. White women were much more likely than other groups to be diagnosed with Borderline Personality Disorder.

DEVELOPMENT OF THE PROJECT

Initial Assessment

In addition to the comprehensive description of the women in the target population, the project conducted an extensive process evaluation which commenced with a needs assessment in District 14, followed by focus groups, interviews with 59 agency program managers and direct care staff, chart reviews of 200 clients of the lead agency, and 10 in-depth case studies. These multiple methods provided rich information about the existing treatment system, service needs, and barriers faced by women with co-occurring disorders in this study and was used to inform the development of the Triad interventions.

Survey information from the key informants was collected using the service delivery questionnaire developed by Morrissey et al. (1994) for the National Evaluation of the Demonstration Program for the Chronically Mentally Ill. Key informant ratings of the adequacy, quality, availability and coordination of services were compared to results reported by Morrissey et al. (1997) for one urban and one rural county in North Carolina. Results indicated that while there was already some communication and cooperation among agencies, there was a need for increased coordination of services and large service gaps.

At the beginning of the Triad Women's Project, services in the District included a full continuum of mental health and AOD services for adults and children provided by two primary mental health agencies and one AOD agency, Tri-County Human Services (TCHS), which was also the lead agency.

Focus groups were held in the Tri-County area in order to gather information from consumer/survivor/recovery (CSRs) persons on what services were available to them in the targeted area and what changes and improvements they recommend for these services. Their feedback highlighted the importance of transportation, housing, employment, and parenting skills. Three gaps were identified by CSRs: housing for women and children, therapy groups for women only that focused on abuse issues, and transportation The secondary focus of the meetings was to begin involvement of CSRs on all levels of the Triad Project. Many of the women at these initial meetings became involved directly in the project as Consumer Advisory Board members, advocates and consultants.

Developing Interventions

From our developmental research and a review of the research and practice literature, it was clear that three services were needed to better serve the target population: (1) an integrated, intensive case management model, (2) an innovative and easily transportable group model that fully integrates mental health, AOD, and trauma issues and blends psychoeducational and process methods, and (3) integrated, peer-run services that empower survivors. All these services were to be gender-specific and include a focus on parenting.

The Triad interventions were developed based on empirical evidence and follow the conceptual work of many (Drake, McHugo, & Noordsy, 1993; Harris, 1996; Drake, Mueser, Clark, & Wallach, 1996; Jerrell & Ridgely, 1995; Minkoff, 1997; Stein & Santos, 1998; Bassuk, Melnick, & Browne, 1998; Rapp, 1997). These researchers have documented the importance of intensive, team- and strengths-based case management for people with co-occurring disorders, and the effectiveness of skills-oriented, psychoeducational groups for decreasing mental health, AOD, and trauma-related problems.

The Triad Women's Project formed the Clinical Interventions Committee that included trauma specialists, AOD providers, people in recovery, mental health providers, consumers of mental health services, experts in co-occurring disorders, and research team members. The committee began its work by developing a consensus on treatment principles and further articulating the underlying philosophy of the development and course of co-occurring disorders and the impact of violence on the lives of these women. As can be imagined, each of the members had their own, frequently divergent, views. Hours of listening, discussion, reading, writing and revising went into building a consensus that reflected all voices. The resulting document of the philosophical basis for our interventions was reviewed and sanctioned by the Consumer Advisory Board and the Triad Council.

The case managers, or resource coordination and advocacy providers were given the title "Triad Specialists" and the group was named the Triad Group for their attention to all three issues: mental health, AOD, and trauma.

The Triad Women's Groups (Clark & Fearday, 2003) were derived and expanded from existing integrated, trauma-specific, and gender-specific group models provided at the Florida Center for Addictions and Dual Disorders and the Residential Assessment and Stabilization Unit for Women in Tri-County Human Services, which have been providing groups for many years to women with dual disorders who have survived violence. The Group model also drew from these works: *Trauma Recovery and Empowerment* by Maxine Harris (1998); *Treating Addicted Survivors of Trauma* by Evans and Sullivan (1995); *Skills Training Manual for Treating Borderline Personality Disorder* by Marsha Linehan (1993); and *Therapy for Adults Molested as Children* by John Briere (1996). While based on sound research, the resulting intervention is unique.

The Clinical Interventions Committee drafted the group model and wrote the Triad Group manual (Clark, 2002). The principles and statement on the impact of violence are frequently referred to in this manual and underlie the group intervention.

We also conducted a pilot study of the Triad experimental group intervention. The study examined pre- and post-intervention data on 128 women who participated in the experimental group treatment. Although not conclusive, as no comparison was made with women not receiving the Triad Group, a few interesting findings emerged. First, as measured by the Coping Responses Inventory (CRI) (Moos, 1997), there was an increase in adaptive coping skills (i.e., approach behaviors) and a decrease in the less constructive "avoidance behaviors" associated with alcohol and other drug abuse and trauma reactions. There was also a decrease in mental health symptoms as measured by the Brief Symptom Inventory (Derogatis, 1993). Only one subgroup of women, those with few trauma related symptoms at baseline as measured by the Trauma Symptom Checklist-40 (Elliot & Briere, 1992), failed to show improvement on the pilot study outcome measures for the Triad groups. Piloting of the group intervention and findings from the pre- and post-tests and chart reviews of all pilot groups participants were fed back to the committee developing the group intervention.

A smaller group of the Clinical Interventions Committee developed the Triad Specialist model. Triad Specialist activities were designed to assess and address the service needs of the target population. A careful review of existing case management services in the district was done. The challenge for this component was to identify methods of enhancing and integrating existing services to better meet population needs and yet continue to be feasible in the existing system. The Wisconsin Quality of Life Instrument (WQLI) (Becker, Diamond, & Sainfort, 1993) was added as part of the intervention to enhance the working alliance and negotiated goal setting. The WQLI includes consumer and provider ratings of the importance of, and current functioning in, several quality of life domains and goals for treatment.

Triad Specialists were trained to assist women across service delivery settings and systems and address barriers to services by participating on the Triad Team, a group of Triad Specialists, Triad Group facilitators, and clinical consultants that meet biweekly in rotating locations throughout the district. Piloting of the Triad Specialist intervention and findings from the pre- and post-tests of all pilot Triad Specialist participants was fed back to the committee developing and implementing the clinical case management intervention. The Triad Specialist intervention was also manualized.

Consumer Advisory Board members expressed their need for a Peer Support Group. Women that graduated from the sixteen-week Triad Group stated that they needed peer support in order to continue healing from trauma issues. They needed somewhere safe to share what happened to them and to be heard. They wanted to learn more about how trauma affected their lives and wanted support in changing their behaviors. They wanted to be in the company of other trauma survivors and hear of their experience, strength and hope. CSRs along with consultants developed the Wisdom of Women peer support group.

Three consumer leaders in the project designed the peer support group activities. One woman had extensive experience developing groups and Internet supports for survivors of violence. The second woman was in recovery and had extensive experience with the 12-step community. The third consumer leader is a nationally known consumer and advocate of mental health services. Their combined efforts resulted in the development of the Wisdom of Women (WOW) peer-run groups.

Triad Specialists, Triad Group facilitators, and consumer leaders participated in a fifteen-week training program that addressed counseling skills, gender-specific issues, integrated care, trauma issues, parenting skills, psychiatric medications, ethics, cultural diversity, and available community resources. The one-time training sessions were manualized and videotaped for training new Triad Specialists and Triad Group facilitators.

Developing Services Integration

The focus of the intervention was at the individual level in the form of three new services and on services rather than systems integration. However, a number of coordination activities at the systems level supported the services integration. The agencies had a district-wide planning process and were members of the district's Joint Clinical Committee. They worked to develop and implement the standardized and integrated biopsychosocial assessment across agencies. Psychosocial assessments, including mental health problems, AOD, trauma history, and parenting issues, from several programs and agencies across the system were collected. Given that information, the providers jointly developed a comprehensive biopsychosocial assessment that met the clinicians' need for information and agency requirements of all of their respective funders and accrediting bodies (e.g., Medicaid, Commission on Accreditation of Rehabilitation Facilities [CARF], Joint Commission on Accreditation of Healthcare Organizations [JCAHO]). The motivating force behind this product development was to reduce the number of times a women would have to repeat her life story, especially trauma histories, and that regardless of which "door" she entered, she would get a comprehensive assessment resulting in an integrated services/treatment plan.

The three participating agencies developed memoranda of understanding allowing the sharing of office space; addressed confidentiality issues, and allowed the sharing of records; and permitted flexibility in serving common clients (i.e., no one "owns" a client). A series of collaborative agreements to integrate crisis intervention were implemented. As clients in the psychiatric crisis stabilization unit are identified as having AOD issues, AOD liaison staff are notified and visit the clients for further assessment and arrange for AOD services as requested by the client. The same process is initiated for clients in the detox unit who request mental health services or are assessed as having mental health issues. One of the liaison staff has been trained as a Triad group facilitator. The agencies continued to be autonomous, but resources were shared and there was joint planning and collaboration.

The Triad Council is a district-wide committee including the agencies providing Triad Services, but also other providers and stakeholders throughout the area. Initially the Triad Council was comprised of staff and consumers directly involved in the project and served as an organizational and coordinating group for the developmental phase. This function was later taken over by a smaller steering committee of service administrators, a research liaison and consumer leaders. The Triad Council became a forum for the all agencies in the community that work in some way with women and their children similar to the target population. The Council contributed in large part to developing a trauma-informed service system in the district.

DESCRIPTION OF THE INTERVENTIONS

Philosophy and Principles

Each of the interventions is based on the philosophy and principles developed by the Clinical Interventions Committee. One of the primary hypotheses underlying this project is that integrated treatment for mental health disorders, AOD, and trauma will be more effective than treatment that addresses these problems separately. Service systems present barriers when they require women with these problems to seek services from various agencies and individuals. These barriers can be particularly difficult for women living in poverty, lacking affordable housing, raising children, and lacking transportation. The often unrecognized traumatizing effects of violence on the lives of women, such as low self-esteem, impaired trust, shame, and anxiety, raise the height of these barriers.

The principles of recovery, empowerment, and survival emphasize positive outcomes for women. Other principles that articulate the project's philosophies and underlie treatment for women with Triad issues include integrated services, flexibility, readiness, strength-based assessment and treatment, self-help, trauma-informed services, gender-specific services cultural sensitivity, and confidentiality.

Readiness: the acceptance of help for problems related to mental illness, AOD, and violence occurs for women in different degrees and stages. Ongoing assessment of a woman's readiness is needed to provide a correct fit between readiness and intervention efforts.

Flexibility: to provide individualized attention to the needs of CSR women so that treatment addresses the diverse preferences and needs of the women receiving services. Flexibility reflects an attitude of collaboration between staff and clients.

Strength-based assessment and treatment: to identify what women do well and how they have coped with disempowering environments. Of equal importance is identifying positive support and care available in women's environments. It is vital that assessments focus on a woman's resilience, skills, life goals, and hopes for the future.

Self-help: the process of CSR women helping other CSR women is a powerful tool for recovery. CSR women have powerful stories to share with each other. When one CSR woman shares her recovery story with another, both women are helped.

Trauma-informed services: to provide services that reflect an understanding of the complex impact of trauma on the lives of survivors. Attention is given to survivor safety and the development of collaborative, trusting relationships. Goals of treatment focus on growth, mastery, and efficacy rather than on the absence of symptoms.

Gender-specific services: to provide services that are designed to meet the unique needs and strengths of women. Services must recognize and respect the value women place on interdependency, nurturing relationships, and the communication of feelings.

Cultural sensitivity: the quality or condition of being capable of perceiving and respecting a woman's ethnicity when providing outreach, assessment and treatment.

In addition, the committee developed two statements reflecting the consensus of the group, current research, and best practice guidelines. The first was on the development and course of co-occurring disorders emphasizing their interrelation and the need for integrated services. The second statement dealt with the impact of violence on the development and course of co-occurring disorders emphasizing the centrality of trauma and the importance of both considering trauma in all services and providing trauma-specific services.

Group Therapy

The Triad Women's Group therapy model is built upon four-phases. It runs 16 weeks, two hours per session and has open enrollment. In *Phase I: Mindfulness*, the concept of an integrated, safe, and supportive group for women with co-occurring disorders is introduced, and women begin an exploration of the connections between healing the effects of trauma and recovery and mental health. They acquire personal empowerment, skills for maintaining their safety and develop awareness of their choices regarding their thoughts and feelings. *Phase II: Interpersonal Effectiveness and Skills* addresses the relational aspects of living and growing with Triad issues. In *Phase III: Emotional Regulation*, women build specific skills such as self-soothing and dealing effectively with cravings and urges, and they move toward understanding their issues at a spiritual level. Finally, in *Phase IV: Distress Tolerance*, women practice skills to manage the most challenging aspects of living with and overcoming alcoholism and drug abuse, trauma and mental illness, such as dealing with violence and crisis management.

The group model is structured to promote productive use of the time and to maximize skill building with some time designated for education about the connections between trauma, AOD problems, and mental illness and with strategies for coping and empowerment. Flexibility in the use of open discussion and sharing during a portion of the group is maintained to permit women to draw support from the group no matter where they might be in the recovery process. This combination of structure and flexibility provides a sense of safety that women can get their needs met and that boundaries will be respected, while honoring that women enter the group with remarkable strength and knowledge. Training for the implementation of the Triad Women's Group is through a co-facilitation model in which a Triad-trained staff member or consultant runs the group in cooperation with a program-based counselor for up to the complete 16 weeks. New Triad Women's Group facilitators are typically counselors in mental health or AOD treatment settings, both inpatient and outpatient. All are female and have some additional knowledge concerning women's or trauma services, and all had a special interest in serving women with Triad issues.

Many women have commented that they felt more hopeful and supported after participating in the group, that they felt much less alone after learning that other women had experiences like theirs; that the Triad Women's Group felt safer, a better fit, or more compatible with their needs than other therapies they had experienced. Provider responses were similarly positive. An outpatient mental health program director noted that the Triad Women's Group improved his site's overall group attendance rates. A number of Triad Women's Groups are currently operating in a variety of AOD treatment, mental health, residential, and outpatient settings in the district.

Resource Coordination and Advocacy

The Triad Specialist model of clinical case management, resource coordination, and advocacy can be characterized by four principles, including trauma informed service provision, integrated mental health and AOD services, continuity of care, and advocacy.

Trauma informed service provision: Triad Specialists are prepared to assist women with identifying and relieving trauma symptoms, and to support them as they move through experiences in recovery that could be retraumatizing. Training on the effects of childhood physical abuse, childhood sexual abuse, domestic violence, and rape, as well as strategies for supporting the healing process are included in the Triad Specialist training series and additional training in this area is provided by the Trauma Clinical Trainer on an ongoing basis.

Services integrated for mental health and AOD problems: Triad Specialists typically work in either AOD treatment or mental health settings, so all are cross-trained in these care models, and educated about the benefits of integrated care. The Triad Team consists of providers from mental health and AOD treatment programs and CSRs. The Triad Team is also a source of referral information. Triad Specialists bridge gaps between agencies and service paradigms by communicating in the Triad Team, attending training at various agencies, building awareness, and regularly contacting other agencies and programs regarding the women they served.

Continuity of care: This is a unique aspect of the Triad Specialist role, especially in AOD treatment settings. That contact is maintained and care is provided after the woman leaves the primary care setting. Triad Specialists commit to serving women on their caseloads for at least one year, or longer if the woman wishes to continue services. This continuity of care bridges service gaps and prevents women from "falling through the cracks." This commitment acknowledges that relapse, decompensation, or crisis is occasionally part of the overall recovery process, particularly for women with the many and complex challenges related to co-occurring disorders and violence, and the outcome is better when support is available through difficult times as well as when women make upward progress. Many women return to services when they may not have otherwise because of the ongoing support of their Triad Specialists.

Advocacy-Triad Specialists interact with organizations on behalf of women and their children to minimize barriers to goal attainment. For example, the child protection, shelter, and reunification processes in the

Department of Children and Families often seems overwhelming to women, and Triad Specialists assist mothers in negotiating these processes by providing referrals to services required in their reunification plans, documenting progress toward reunification goals, and accompanying them to court. Triad Specialists similarly advocate for women involved in the criminal justice system, suggest treatment in sentencing recommendations, and increase women's access to services from jail and prison.

Attendance at the aforementioned Triad Team is one of the functions of Triad Specialists. It is a source of peer supervision, training, and support for Triad Specialists, Triad Women's Group Facilitators, CSR staff, and consultants. It meets every other week at rotating locations in the district. In the Triad Team meetings providers of Triad services receive training and technical assistance from experts in the field in skill areas such as active listening, provider self-care, strategies for serving women with dissociative disorders, addressing codependency, and crisis intervention. Triad Specialists assist one another in the Triad Team by sharing about service resources and treatment strategies, address service needs of women on their caseloads, and also support their agencies by billing their service-related activities there. Other Triad Specialist functions include completing the WQLI with women for goal planning and negotiation, service linking, and maintaining their skill levels in training. It was determined that in order to effectively serve women with Triad issues, caseload sizes should be kept down to 25 for full-time Triad Specialists, and contacts with women in need of active service participation should occur at least once per week, preferably face-to-face.

The Consumer Advisory Board

The mission of the Consumer Advisory Board is to educate and empower participants regarding consumer issues. Members endeavor to effect policy change regarding consumer choice in services and also to contribute consumer perspective for the Triad Project. The Consumer Advisory Board has had input into the Women, Co-occurring Disorders and Violence Study Grant application, the baseline interview, the Triad Group model and Wisdom of Women peer support group. The Consumer Advisory Board is comprised of women who are in recovery from alcoholism and drug abuse, mental illness and have experienced trauma in their lives. They are women in treatment and services, they come from the 12-Step recovery community, and are graduates of the Program. The graduates give the women in treatment hope that they can recover too. The meetings are held monthly for two hours in various locations throughout the Tri-County area in order to make them accessible to members in treatment. CSRs are paid a stipend of $10.00 for attending and travel reimbursement for those who drive.

The agenda is prepared by the Consumer Coordinator based on the specific needs of the consumers. For example, the Program Director of Winter Haven Hospital presented on Florida's Assertive Community Treatment teams and discussed his Agency's consumer integration; a leading consumer advocate of the Boston Consortium of Services for Families in Recovery presented a leadership development training; a woman in a 12-Step recovery program and WOW group participant shared her "Story"; a founding Consumer Advisory Board member and consumer advocate presented on mental illness and we viewed a video she produced called "Stigma"; and a psychologist and parenting expert presented on addressing children's and parents' needs throughout the process of separation and reunification.

Peer Support Group

The peer support group, Wisdom of Women (WOW), has proven very popular. The peer services model integrates some 12-Step principles, strategies for effective coping with mental health issues such as PTSD, and support for healing the effects of trauma. Unique to the model are goals for empowerment known as "The Five S's": Safety, Serenity, Sense of Self, Support System, and Solving Life's Problems. The Peer Services Committee developed a "starter kit" for women with a brochure, principles, group guidelines, preamble and pertinent information regarding co-dependence, abuse, PTSD, developing boundaries, etc. Education is a key component of the WOW group.

Each peer group leader has a job description and participates in a formal training. The WOW group model is a vital addition to the care continuum, providing support to women completing treatment in the Triad Women's Group, and presenting an opportunity for support for women who may not feel comfortable in traditional care settings or in 12-Step meetings. It is welcoming to women in that it is free of charge and confidential. WOW has demonstrated to the provider community that while professional help may be beneficial (and sometimes not), women with trauma and other issues can as a group heal themselves. WOW groups operate in community sites scattered around the large district for easy accessibility.

The groups are led by Consumers and have specific guidelines and a model that they follow. There are currently five Wisdom of Women groups throughout the Tri-County area. We also have attracted women who have been or are affected by sexual or physical abuse in their lives. Victim Advocates have referred many victims of domestic violence to WOW. Fortunately, we have been able to fill a service gap. We are hoping in the future to bring WOW to incarcerated women with trauma issues.

Parenting Intervention

Triad Specialist services are parenting informed. The majority of women served in the project are mothers, and Triad Specialists recognize the importance of the well-being of children to mothers in recovery. Project participants have commented on how the potential of harm to or for loss of their children motivated them for recovery, and how the stress of losing custody of their children greatly exacerbated their AOD problems or mental illness. A child development and childhood trauma expert sits as a consultant on the Triad Team, and Triad Specialists receive ongoing training on parenting issues. The parenting and child development consultant provides training on topics such as the effects of maternal mental illness, AOD problems, and trauma histories on child development; assisting mothers in the shelter and reunification processes, supporting the healing of children who are victims or witnesses of violence, and assisting mothers with Triad issues to advocate for their children. The parenting and child development consultant highlights the strengths and resiliencies of child and adult survivors of trauma. It is part of the role of Triad Specialist to refer each woman on her caseload to parenting classes, and progress on parenting goals is discussed in Triad Specialist contacts with women in the intervention.

Triad Specialists were also trained to encourage women to attend one of the three models of parenting classes available in the district: Systematic Training for Effective Parenting (STEP) classes; Parenting Tools for Positive Behavior Change; and the Nurturing Program for Families. In addition, a *Staff Handbook for Addressing Parenting Needs* (Kuehnle & Becker, 2001) and a *Handbook for Triad Mothers* (Kuehnle & Becker, 2001) were written and distributed to support both Triad Specialists and parents in their efforts to improve parenting skills. In addition to providing information relevant to parenting skills these manuals provided information about the Dependency Court system and its operations.

Lessons Learned

By combining so many voices from a complex community in this venture, we were able to learn many lessons that may apply to other settings. For one, to successfully develop and implement a project such as this requires persistent effort over an extended period of time. A great deal of time is needed to develop communication channels and build consensus. In addition, these women's lives have multiple layers and the recovery work requires a long-term commitment.

Consistently, we saw the importance of developing services that can "fit" into the existing system and be billable. Additional funds were necessary to reimburse agencies for lost billable hours while staff attended meetings to develop the interventions. Were these agency staff not available to participate in the development of the interventions, implementation of the new services would have been impeded. However, once developed, to be maintained and sustained they must utilize and even maximize existing resources, however scarce.

The application of evidence-based practices and the implementation of new modalities in a district's service system must also accommodate the system's existing realities. Research and new service implementation must be fit into current practice and woven into routine procedures, and not imposed. Similarly, the services must fit and be responsive to the environment. In a semi-rural, low population density area such as this, transportation is a vital concern. Behavioral and physical healthcare services, jobs, childcare, even socialization are limited by the lack of public transportation and the expense of private transportation. To ignore such factors means a failure of service delivery.

AOD agencies are, in general, not familiar with case management and a number of adjustments to policies and procedures were needed to implement this. Working with this population can be quite stressful and the Triad team has become a major source of support for the Triad specialists. Unfortunately, group facilitators expressed disappointment in the lack of similar support and opportunities to problem solve. The project was designed to have the facilitators also attend Triad team meetings; however, their "missed time" was too expensive for agencies since they could not bill for it. In addition, the fact that staff often had to travel some distance to attend the meetings was also an expense.

Continued collaboration with these women has demonstrated the importance of the relationship or therapeutic alliance when working together. This has reinforced the importance of a clinical case management model rather than the linking/brokering model of some systems. Resources and services are scarce and often inaccessible. To simply refer someone to another agency would be inadequate.

Systems respond in predictable ways to the prospect of change in practice and service philosophy. There seems universally to be a significant initial resistance. Taking the time to build consensus among key stakeholders was a good investment and helped tremendously with innovation "buy-in." Awareness building and demonstrating success with new interventions, such as with the Triad Women's and WOW groups appear to promote support and foster increased communication with and between agencies (Clark, Giard, & Becker, 2003).

Lastly, it has been harder to integrate CSRs into agencies than initially thought. While there appears to be a commitment to listening to the CSR voice and responding, for example, to advocacy issues raised, there have been a number of barriers to having consumers in position of power. AOD agencies have a long history of having people in recovery on their boards, but difficulties arise when that person has been served by that same agency. Similar problems and issues of confidentiality were raised in mental health agencies. The project continues to work on these issues.

Conclusions

The Triad Women's Project successfully implemented three gender-specific, trauma-informed, and integrated services in rural Florida for women with co-occurring mental health and AOD disorders and histories of trauma. The three services, case management, group therapy, and peer-run groups, also addressed parenting issues as most of the women have children. The needs assessment and developmental and implementation processes included CSR involvement at every level and all phases of the project confirmed the critical importance of designing services with the above ingredients. Successful efforts like this one require time, consensus-building, consumer involvement, and support for direct care staff.

REFERENCES

Bassuk, E.L., Melnick, S., & Browne, A. (1998). Responding to the needs of low income and homeless women who are survivors of family violence. *Journal of the American Medical Women's Association, 53*(2), 57-64.

Becker, M., Diamond, R., & Sainfort, F. (1993). A new client centered index for measuring quality of life in persons with severe and persistent mental illness. *Quality of Life Research, 2*(4), 239-251.

Briere, J. (1996). *Therapy for adults molested as children.* New York: Springer.

Bureau of Economic and Business Research. (1999). *Florida statistical abstract: 1999.* Gainesville: University of Florida.

Carey, K.B. (1996). Treatment of co-occurring AOD and major mental illness. In R.E. Drake & K.T. Mueser (Eds.), *New directions for mental health services* (pp. 19-31). San Francisco: Jossey-Bass.

Clark, C. & Fearday, F. (Eds.). (2003). *Triad Women's Project: Group facilitator's manual.* Tampa, FL: University of South Florida. Manuscript submitted for publication.

Clark, C., Giard, J., & Becker, M. (2003, February). Developing and evaluating integrated services for women. Paper presented at the 13th Annual Conference on State Mental Health Agency Services Research, Program Evaluation, and Policy, Baltimore.

Clark, C. (2002, November). The Triad Women's Project. Paper presented at the International Society for the Study of Dissociative Disorders 19th International Fall Conference, Baltimore.

Derogatis, L.R. (1993). *Brief Symptom Inventory (BSI) administration, scoring, and procedures manual.* (3rd ed.). Minneapolis, MN: National Computer Systems.

Drake, R.E., McHugo, G.J., & Noordsy, D.L. (1993). Treatment of alcoholism among schizophrenic outpatients: 4-year outcomes. *American Journal of Psychiatry, 150*(2), 328-329.

Drake, R.E., Mueser, K.T., Clark, R.E., & Wallach, M.A. (1996). The course, treatment, and outcome of substance disorder in persons with severe mental illness. *American Journal of Orthopsychiatry, 66*(1), 42-51.

Elliot, D.M. & Briere, J. (1992). Sexual abuse trauma among professional women: Validating the Trauma Symptom Checklist-40 (TSC-40). *Child Abuse and Neglect, 16*, 391-398.

Evans, K. & Sullivan, J.M. (1995). *Treating addicted survivors of trauma.* New York: Guilford Press.

Harris, M. (1998). *Trauma recovery and empowerment.* New York: The Free Press.

Harris, M. (1996). Treating sexual abuse trauma with dually diagnosed women. *Community Mental Health Journal, 32*, 371-385.

Jerrell, J.M. & Ridgely, M.S. (1995). Gender differences in the assessment of specialized treatments for AOD among people with severe mental illness. *Journal of Psychoactive Drugs, 27*, 347-355.

Kuehnle, K. & Becker, M. (2001). *Handbook for Triad mothers.* Tampa: University of South Florida.

Kuehnle, K. & Becker, M. (2001). *Staff handbook for addressing parenting needs.* Tampa: University of South Florida.

Linehan, M.M. (1993). *Cognitive-behavioral treatment of borderline personality disorder.* New York: The Guilford Press.

Minkoff, K. (1997). Integration of addiction and psychiatric treatment. In N.S. Miller & J. Fine (Eds.), *The principles and practice of addictions in psychiatry* (pp. 191-199). Philadelphia: Saunders.

Moos, R.H. (1997). Assessing approach and avoidance coping skills and their determinants and outcomes. *Indian Journal of Clinical Psychology, 24*(1), 58-64.

Morrissey, J.P., Calloway, M., Bartko, W.T., Ridgely, M.S., Goldman, H.H., & Paulson, R.I. (1994). Local mental health authorities and service system change: Evidence from the Robert Wood Johnson program on chronic mental illness. *The Milbank Quarterly, 72*(1), 49-80.

Morrissey, J.P., Calloway, M., Johnsen, M., & Ullman, M. (1997). Service system performance and integration: A baseline profile of the ACCESS demonstration sites. *Psychiatric Services, 48*(3), 374-380.

Office of Program Policy Analysis and Government Accountability. (1999). *Justification review: Alcohol, drug abuse and mental health program (Report 99-09).* Tallahassee, FL: Author.

Rapp, C.A. (1997). *The strengths model.* New York: Oxford University Press.

Ridgely, M., Goldman, H., & Willenbring, M. (1990). Barriers to the care or persons with dual diagnosis: Organizational and financial issues. *Schizophrenia Bulletin, 16* (1), 123-132.

Ridgely, M.S., Lambert, D., Goodman, A., Chichester, C.S., & Ralph, R. (1998). Interagency collaboration in services for people with co-occurring mental illness and substance use disorder. *Psychiatric Services, 49*(2), 236-238.

State of Florida Agency for Health Care Administration (AHCA). (1999). *Drug abuse hospitalization costs study.* Tallahassee, FL: Author.

Stein, L.I. & Santos, A.B. (1998). *Assertive community treatment of persons with severe mental illness.* New York: Norton.

Zweben, J. (1996). Psychiatric problems among alcohol and other drug dependent women. *Journal of Psychiatric Drugs, 28*(4), 345-366.

The Women Embracing Life and Living (WELL) Project: Using the Relational Model to Develop Integrated Systems of Care for Women with Alcohol/Drug Use and Mental Health Disorders with Histories of Violence

Norma Finkelstein, PhD
Laurie S. Markoff, PhD

SUMMARY. Based on the relational model of women's development, WELL Project interventions include Integrated Care Facilitators providing resource coordination and advocacy services, *Seeking Safety* trauma groups, *Nurturing Families Affected by Substance Abuse, Mental Illness and Trauma* parenting groups, and *WELL Recovery*, a self/mutual help group for women with co-occurring disorders and trauma. Interventions were delivered at three agencies licensed to provide substance abuse and mental health services, impacting three communities. In preparation, consumers, providers and policymakers met in Local Leadership Councils in each community and in a State Leadership Council, participating

Norma Finkelstein and Laurie S. Markoff are both affiliated with the WELL Project.

[Haworth co-indexing entry note]: "The Women Embracing Life and Living (WELL) Project: Using the Relational Model to Develop Integrated Systems of Care for Women with Alcohol/Drug Use and Mental Health Disorders with Histories of Violence." Finkelstein, Norma, and Laurie S. Markoff. Co-published simultaneously in *Alcoholism Treatment Quarterly* (The Haworth Press, Inc.) Vol. 22, No. 3/4, 2004, pp. 63-80; and: *Responding to Physical and Sexual Abuse in Women with Alcohol and Other Drug and Mental Disorders: Program Building* (ed: Bonita M. Veysey, and Colleen Clark) The Haworth Press, Inc., 2004, pp. 63-80. Single or multiple copies of this article are available for a fee from The Haworth Document Delivery Service [1-800-HAWORTH, 9:00 a.m. - 5:00 p.m. (EST). E-mail address: docdelivery@haworthpress.com].

in cross-training and collaborative discussions planning for integrated, trauma-informed care. *[Article copies available for a fee from The Haworth Document Delivery Service: 1-800-HAWORTH. E-mail address: <docdelivery@ haworthpress.com> Website: <http://www.HaworthPress.com> © 2004 by The Haworth Press, Inc. All rights reserved.]*

KEYWORDS. Alcoholism, drug abuse, women, physical abuse, sexual abuse, state

INTRODUCTION

The Institute for Health and Recovery (IHR), based in Cambridge, Massachusetts, is a statewide non-profit organization focused on the populations of families with alcohol and other drug (AOD) abuse and/or co-occurring disorders. IHR provides systems, policy and program development aimed at designing and developing services for families, especially women and their children. IHR takes as its theoretical basis the relational model developed by the Stone Center at Wellesley College (Finkelstein, 1996; Jordan et al., 1991; Markoff & Cawley, 1996). This model, which emphasizes the role of relationship in the lives of women and in bringing about change, informed and shaped the design of IHR's project to address the needs of women with co-occurring disorders and histories of violence, the WELL Project.

STATEMENT OF THE PROBLEM

The overarching goal of the Women, Co-Occurring Disorders and Violence Project (WCDV) is to test the hypothesis that trauma-informed, integrated services will lead to better outcomes than services as usual for women with co-occurring disorders and histories of violence and their children. During the first two years of the project, representatives from different sites across the county worked together to design the outcome study and to make decisions about the defining parameters of the intervention model. Individual sites would be able to choose an intervention model that fit their particular context within those parameters.

Each site, therefore, used the first two years of the project to design the interventions and the intervention model to be used in the second phase of the project. However, it was believed that it was not sufficient to simply provide trauma-informed, integrated interventions; the service delivery system itself must be changed in order to support such interventions. Providing a trauma intervention could actually have a negative effect if the agency in which it is delivered was not trauma-informed (Harris & Fallot, 2001). For example, a woman might become triggered in a trauma group and choose to leave the group in order to ground herself. This attempt at self-care might be responded to in a punitive way in a setting in which "leaving group" is considered a rule infraction. By the same token, providing concurrent mental health and AOD abuse services, even in the same agency, can be detrimental if the underlying philosophies of the providers are not the same and women get conflicting messages about the best way to proceed. To avoid these pitfalls, it was necessary to spend the first two years of the project working to prepare the service delivery system for the delivery of trauma-informed, integrated care.

In Massachusetts, services are primarily funded directly by the state. For example, there is no county-based system of health/human services funding. Therefore, changes in the service delivery system are usually best brought about by working at the state level. Because the WELL Project was expected to eventually impact the entire service delivery system, it was designed to have a statewide focus. At the same time, services are delivered at the local community level, and communities differ in their makeup and their needs. Therefore, the WELL Project was implemented at three local sites, intending to impact three local communities. These local sites were three large, comprehensive private non-profit organizations licensed to provide both mental health and AOD abuse services: CAB Health and Recovery (CAB) in Northeast Massachusetts, Gosnold on Cape Cod and the Islands, and Stanley Street Treatment and Resources (SSTAR) in Fall River. In addition, two sites were participants in a Children's Sub-Study, the WELL Child Project. A fourth site, Spectrum Health Systems, Inc., in Worcester, served as the Comparison site, and did not receive WELL Project interventions. All four sites were historically established to treat AOD abuse, offering a complete continuum of AOD abuse treatment services: (i.e., detoxification, residential and outpatient). Within the last few years, mental health outpatient and residential services have been added.

Although both mental health and AOD services were available at sites prior to implementation of the WELL Project, the degree to which they were integrated varied. Only one site provided an integrated assessment that could result in both a substance abuse and mental health diagnosis. All three intervention sites had some dual diagnosis services;

one site was in the process of establishing a dual diagnosis detoxification program, and another site had a dual diagnosis residential program.

Services for women experiencing domestic violence were available in all three communities, but were not integrated into mental health and AOD treatment. One site did have its own Women's Center that provided domestic violence counseling and advocacy and this made them more sensitive to issues of violence. For example, they were the only site that did ask about histories of abuse in their intake. Two of the sites also at times had conducted trauma groups; however, no attempt was made to assess or address trauma for women who requested AOD abuse or mental health services. Community providers of violence services did not assess for AOD and mental health problems. If such problems were known to exist for a particular client, violence providers would often refer the client out to AOD or mental health treatment providers because they did not feel they could meet their needs.

At the state level, funding streams for mental health, AOD and violence services are separate, which has resulted historically in treatment being provided in a parallel, non-integrated fashion. Some attempts at integrating AOD and mental health services were being made prior to the beginning of the WELL Project. The Massachusetts Department of Mental Health had received an Exemplary Practice grant from SAMHSA to create a Community Consensus-Building Collaborative to develop strategies for integrating AOD and mental health services. The contractor responsible for managing behavioral health funds for Medicaid had contracted with the Peer Educators Project of Vinfen, Inc., a comprehensive mental health agency, to develop "Double Trouble" Twelve Step self-help groups for individuals with co-occurring AOD and mental health disorders. Some attempts were also being made to meet the needs of women with both domestic violence and AOD problems. Two residential programs for these women and their children had been funded by the Department of Social Services and were in the start-up phase of implementation. However, for the most part, the AOD abuse, mental health and trauma service delivery systems were not integrated.

It was the task of the WELL Project to create a context at the agency, community and state levels that would support the delivery of trauma-informed, integrated services. This involved developing or enhancing linkages among state agencies and among provider organizations, educating provider organizations so that they could integrate an understanding of trauma into their services, and selecting the interventions to be used in the study.

PROGRAM MANAGEMENT STRUCTURE

IHR was the lead agency on the project and contracted with Health and Addictions Research, Inc. for project evaluation. The project was administered by a Project Steering Committee, which consisted of the Principal Investigator, Project Director, Project Research Director from Health and Addictions Research, administrators from each of the local sites and two consumer representatives. The WELL Project hired a Consumer Coordinator in March of 2000, who joined the Steering Committee at that time.

The Project Director supervised Integrated Care Facilitators (ICFs) who were housed at the three intervention sites. During the first phase of the project, these ICFs, Masters level clinicians knowledgeable about AOD, mental health, and trauma, were responsible for preparing the sites for the delivery of trauma-informed, integrated care. During the second phase they became responsible for delivering and/or supervising the integrated interventions.

PREPARING FOR THE DELIVERY OF TRAUMA-INFORMED, INTEGRATED CARE

Integration of services can only be accomplished within a service system that supports such changes (Minkoff, 2001). Integrating services requires change at the state, community and agency levels of the service system. Using the relational model, the WELL Project worked to bring about change by developing relationships, establishing linkages and working collaboratively with all stakeholders (i.e., consumers, providers, policymakers, advocacy organizations, clinical experts) to determine the best strategies and mechanisms for the delivery of integrated services.

Developing the Cross-Training Curriculum

IHR convened a group of experts called the Expert Resource Panel to provide clinical input into the intervention model and to develop and deliver cross-training for all stakeholders. As these experts began to interact, it became clear that even among professionals who had long histories of working in women's treatment, differences in points of view existed based on training and history of the discipline with which each was primarily identified. To work with this, the group decided to engage in a values clarification exercise conducted by an outside facilitator. When this was accomplished, the group was able to produce a statement of principles, which could then be used to guide the development and delivery of the training curriculum.

In order to achieve integration of services, service providers and policymakers must have basic knowledge of the core content within the fields to be integrated (Cramer, 2001; Minkoff, 2001). Focus groups were conducted with both providers and consumers at each site to identify existing gaps in provider knowledge. Providers were asked what they needed to know in order to be better able to deliver services to women with co-occurring disorders and histories of trauma, and consumers were asked what providers would need to know more about in order to provide better services for them as consumers. Additional focus groups were also conducted with consumers at other AOD abuse treatment programs. These groups focused on what was and was not helpful for the women in treatment, and what products would be useful to help consumers to access appropriate care.

Based on results of these focus groups, a series of training modules were developed. Topics covered included domestic violence, trauma, impact of violence on children, PTSD and AOD, diversity, the trajectory of recovery from multiple issues, gender-specific treatment, and consumer integration. Later, these modules were compiled into a curriculum entitled *WELL Project Training Curriculum for Providers: Developing Integrated Services for Women with Substance Abuse, Mental Illness and Trauma* (Institute for Health and Recovery, 2001). The training based on this curriculum was then provided to the staff of the local sites, to a wider range of providers in the local communities through the Local Leadership Councils (described below) and to policymakers and consumer advocacy organizations through the State Leadership Council (also described below).

Developing Integration at the Agency Level

The primary mechanism for promoting integration at the local sites was the placement of an Integrated Care Facilitator (ICF) at each site. These individuals were employed by the WELL Project to work at and with the sites to move toward an integrated, trauma-informed system of delivering AOD, mental health and violence/trauma services. ICFs attended program and staff meetings, provided input, updated site staff regarding WELL Project activities and participated in case conferences. Their local site participation enabled them to understand and become familiar with the working environment, so they could make informed suggestions regarding changes that might enhance treatment for women and children. They were also the on-site hosts for the cross-training. After approximately one year of cross-training, site representatives to the WELL Project Steering Committee observed that their employees were more knowledgeable about the issues, but were not necessarily able to implement what they had learned. In response, another intervention was developed. This intervention, called "integrated supervision," was provided at each site for two hours each month by one of the clinicians on the WELL Project Expert Resource Panel. Local site clinicians could request a didactic presentation on a relevant topic, discuss challenging cases or discuss systems issues in developing integrated treatment during their integrated supervision time.

Developing Integration at the Community Level

ICFs were also responsible for improving integration of AOD, mental health and violence/trauma services in the community served by the local site. They did this by convening and then chairing a Local Leadership Council (LLC), in which participants could establish or strengthen their relationships and work collaboratively to develop strategies for providing integrated care. These Councils included consumers and representatives from all organizations that might come into contact with a woman with co-occurring disorders and a history of trauma or her children. Having learned from the experience of the Expert Resource Panel, the LLCs began with values clarification. Participants were divided into groups who primarily identified as members of the AOD, mental health or trauma/violence community. Each group was asked to come up with a set of statements about "what is necessary or helpful in order for women with co-occurring disorders and histories of trauma to heal." The facilitator then led a discussion about the similarities and differences between the statements provided by the three groups. This discussion served a number of purposes. Participants were invariably surprised by the similarity of their beliefs, discovering that they viewed the other groups as more different than they actually were. The identified differences were recorded, so that they could be referred to later should disagreement arise. This allowed the source of disagreement to be worked with directly as differences in points of view. It was acknowledged that a diversity of points of view enhanced the creative process, and that everyone concerned wanted to keep the best of the knowledge that had been developed by each of the disciplines.

Following the values clarification process, the LLCs began participating in the cross-training. This would usually consist of one hour of
training, followed by one hour of discussion, led by the ICF. Members
brainstormed the needs of women with co-occurring disorders and histories of trauma and then the needs of the children of such women. Following this, they developed an ideal integrated continuum of care,
maximizing the use of existing resources. This continuum included
components or levels of care and enhancements that would be necessary
in order for existing services to effectively serve this population. These
three continua were eventually combined into one document, the "*Ideal
Integrated Continuum of Care.*" Each LLC then created a service map
that included all existing community services and their contact information. Service maps were compared to the integrated continuum to identify
gaps in service components. From this process, each LLC developed a set
of recommendations, including policy changes that would assist in the integration of care and pilot projects to fill gaps in services. These
recommendations were forwarded to the State Leadership Council (discussed below). Each LLC then chose one recommendation to address lo-
cally. For example, one LLC developed a mechanism for agencies to
continue cross-training each other on an exchange basis. Another LLC
decided to promote universal screening for domestic violence by all service providers in the community. The third LLC decided to develop a
brief document for the community on identifying domestic violence and
developing safety plans.

Developing Integration at the State Level

The mechanism for promoting integration at the state level was the
State Leadership Council (SLC). Convened by IHR, the Council included representatives from a large number of state agencies that serve
women with co-occurring disorders and their children, including the
Department of Public Health/Bureau of Substance Abuse Services, the
Department of Public Health/Sexual Assault Prevention and Survivor
Services, the Department of Mental Health, Department of Social Ser-
vices (Child Protection Agency), the Department of Probation, Office
of Child Care Services and others. Provider advocacy organizations,
such as Jane Doe, Inc. (also known as the Massachusetts Coalition of
Providers of Domestic Violence and Sexual Assault Services) and the
Children's League were included, as well as legislators and consumer
advocacy organizations, such as the Massachusetts Organization for
Addiction Recovery, Parent's Advocacy League and the National Alli-

ance for the Mentally Ill. The Council was chaired by the Principal Investigator of the WELL Project and followed a process similar to that of the LLCs. Cross-training was conducted initially, followed by discussion of the needs of women and their children, and barriers to providing integrated, trauma-informed care.

The SLC accepted the recommendations of the LLCs with minor revisions, and began working on developing and implementing strategies for promoting identified changes. Building on the work of the Expert Resource Panel, the SLC also developed a set of principles to underscore the need for trauma-informed care and outline the specifics of such care. The *Principles for the Trauma-Informed Care of Women with Co-Occurring Mental Health and Substance Abuse Disorders* were drafted in subcommittee and then revised and approved by the SLC. Members of the SLC brought these Principles to their agencies and organizations, asking them to sign a statement of support. To date, 38 organizations have signed such statements, including all of the state agencies principally involved in delivering services to women and children. As a follow-up to this, the SLC developed a WELL Project Tool Kit that includes self-assessments for both provider organizations and state agencies and instructions for using such an assessment to develop an implementation plan to move in the direction of providing trauma-informed, integrated services.

Consumer Integration

In addition to promoting integration of AOD, mental health and violence/trauma services, the WELL Project had as a goal promoting the integration of consumers into service planning and delivery. One means of promoting this was to model it. The WELL Project had consumers in significant numbers on its Steering Committee and on its Local Leadership and State Leadership Councils. For many providers who were members of these Councils, this was a new experience and providers frequently expressed appreciation for this consumer input. However, to integrate consumers successfully, some support services were found to be necessary. Providers needed training regarding the importance of integrating consumers and principles of successful integration. This training was developed by consumers on the Steering Committee with the Project Director and delivered to the local sites. Consumers also needed training on how to be effective advocates. A two-module Leadership Training was developed by consumers on the Steering Committee with the assistance of an expert consumer consultant and delivered to the

WELL Project consumers as a group. Both of these trainings were later included in the *WELL Project Training Curriculum for Providers: Developing Integrated Services for Women with Substance Abuse, Mental Illness and Trauma.*

While consumers actively participated in LLC meetings, they requested time to meet with each other for support and to develop their own advocacy projects. In order to expand these activities and in recognition that consumers on the Steering Committee were volunteers with other full-time jobs, a Consumer Coordinator was hired. The Consumer Coordinator became responsible for recruiting, training, and retaining consumers, for facilitating consumer subcommittees of the LLCs, and for obtaining consumer feedback on all WELL Project procedures and documents.

DELIVERY OF TRAUMA-INFORMED, INTEGRATED SERVICES

Phase II of the WELL Project involved delivering trauma-informed, integrated services at the intervention sites, so that outcomes of women receiving services at those sites could be compared with those of women receiving services as usual at the comparison site. At all four sites, women were screened at intake for AOD abuse, mental health problems, and histories of violence. Women who screened positively in all three areas were offered the opportunity to meet with a research interviewer and could then decide whether or not to participate in the study. Women who chose to participate in the study at the integrated sites were offered the WELL Project interventions.

Women in the Study

In all, 328 women participated in the study, 218 at the intervention sites and 110 at the comparison site. Women ranged in age from 18 to 61, with a mean of 35. Eighty-five percent were White, 8% were African American, 5% were Native American, 1% were Native Hawaiian or other Pacific Islander, and less than 1% were Asian. Seven percent of the women were Latina. The average woman had completed high school. The least educated women had completed seventh grade, while the most educated women had some post-college education. The majority (72%) were not employed. Seventy-one percent of the women had living children under 18, although only 48% were living with one or more of their children upon entering the study.

Eighty-nine percent of the women had been physically abused at some point in their lives. Seventy-four percent had been inappropriately touched or made to touch someone in a sexual way, and 80% had had sex because they felt forced in some way.

In terms of substance abuse, alcohol was the most common drug of choice, accounting for 32% of the women. The average age at first use of alcohol to intoxication was 15, which was the same as average age of first marijuana use. The average age of first use of illegal drugs other than marijuana was slightly older, at age 17. Fifteen percent of the women had used injection drugs in the 30 days prior to the initial interview. Because substance abuse treatment was the point of entry for the study, all women in the study were seeking such treatment upon entry. Of those for whom data is available (264), 65% had prior treatment for alcohol abuse, with an average of 10 starts; 80% had prior treatment for drug abuse, with an average of 12 starts; and 45% had been treated for alcohol and drugs simultaneously, with an average of 9 starts.

Fifty-nine percent of the women had been hospitalized for a psychiatric problem and the average number of hospitalizations was four. The average woman began having mental health problems at age 12. Most women (77%) were receiving mental health services when they entered the study.

Integrating Existing Services

Resource Coordination and Advocacy

Women who chose to participate in the WELL Project were assigned to an ICF, who provided care/resource coordination and advocacy services. According to the relational model, the best context for emotional growth for women is within one or more mutual, empathic, authentic relationships (Jordan et al., 1991; Covington & Surrey, 2000; Miller, 2002). The ICF provided such a connection for each woman, while assisting her in setting goals and accessing services to support her healing. The ICFs followed the women continuously as they moved through the continuum of care, providing the long-term support that trauma survivors often need (Harvey & Harney, 1997). Initially, the ICF conducted a comprehensive interview that covered all aspects of a woman's life: AOD, mental health, trauma (including current safety), relationships (including children), medical, vocational/economic, spiritual and leisure. The ICF then worked collaboratively with the woman to identify areas of her life that she would like to change, setting goals in each area and then prioritizing them. The ICF suggested resources to assist each woman in achieving her goals, including, but not limited to, the integrated interventions discussed below, and helped to address barriers (both internal and external) to accessing those services. Each woman was seen as an expert on her own life and was empowered to make her own choices (Finkelstein, 1994). At the same time, the ICF might help a woman consider the ways in which her trauma, mental illness and AOD abuse interact, and suggest that certain symptoms may have originally developed as a means to cope with trauma, helping the woman to develop a more empowering view of her life experiences. Once an initial integrated service plan was developed, an ICF continued to meet with each woman regularly to assist in overcoming any obstacles to her progress. If a woman was involved with many service providers, the ICF, with the woman's permission, would maintain contact with those providers to ensure that all providers understood her needs in a similar way and that services were coordinated.

Interagency Service Planning

Prior to the intervention phase of the project, subcommittees of the LLCs, called Resource Coordination Councils (RCCs), that included major providers of AOD abuse, mental health and children's services within the local community, met several times to develop plans for interagency referral, information sharing and interagency service planning. These agencies signed Memoranda of Understanding agreeing to participate in this collaborative effort. During the project implementation phase, RCCs continued to meet to discuss progress in integration and to make any needed adjustments to procedures. When necessary, either at a woman's or provider's request, an ICF would convene an interagency service planning meeting with the woman, her treatment providers, and a consumer advocate to address difficulties with the service plan or other barriers to the woman's recovery.

Integrated Interventions

In addition to mechanisms developed to integrate existing services, specific interventions were designed to address AOD, mental illness and trauma simultaneously. Three integrated interventions were made available to women in the WELL Project.

Trauma-Specific Groups

One critical piece was the availability of a group intervention that would help women build skills needed for coping with trauma symptoms, as well as other mental health symptoms and AOD abuse (Bollerud, 1990; Finkelstein et al., 1997; Harris, 1994). Group interventions are particularly helpful as they allow women to develop mutual, authentic, empathic relationships with other women and, in the process, help women to become more empathic with themselves (Fedele & Harrington, 1990). After reviewing and piloting a number of curricula in Phase I, it was decided to use an adapted version of *Seeking Safety* (Najavits, 2002), a curriculum developed by Dr. Lisa Najavits of McClean Hospital and Harvard Medical School, for women with PTSD and AOD abuse. *Seeking Safety* consists of 25 group sessions focused on topics from four content areas: cognitive, behavioral, interpersonal and case management. Najavits and her colleagues (Najavits et al., 1998) reported that the intervention resulted in reductions in AOD use, trauma-related symptoms, suicide risk, and improvements in social adjustment. This curriculum was chosen because it is highly structured, skill-based (rather than uncovering), and directly addresses AOD abuse in every session, making it appropriate even for women in very early recovery. The adaptations involved changes in language to broaden the curriculum to be more inclusive of forms of mental illness other than PTSD, elimination of the case management section as this function was performed by the ICFs, and division of the curriculum into two twelve-session phases. Division of the curriculum was necessary in order to have closed groups and still maintain sufficient numbers of women in each group to be clinically appropriate. When there were drop-outs, women from different phase one groups were combined into a phase two group.

Seeking Safety groups were offered at both residential and outpatient settings. Sessions were either 50 or 75 minutes, based on site constraints. ICFs initially conducted the groups with site clinicians as co-facilitators. As site clinicians became comfortable with the curriculum, they were able to lead groups on their own with ICFs providing supervision.

Parenting Groups

Women are often motivated to seek treatment by the desire to improve the relationships in their lives, particularly relationships with their children (Beckman & Amaro, 1986; Mulford, 1977). Because AOD abuse, mental illness and trauma can have an impact on a woman's ability to parent, an integrated parenting intervention can support women in achieving the goals they define as important in their lives (Lyons-Ruth & Block, 1996; Seval-Brooks & Fitzgerald, 1997; Van Bremen & Chasnoff, 1994). In 1995, IHR adapted Dr. Stephen Bavolek's parenting curriculum, the *Nurturing Program,* creating the *Nurturing Program for Families in Substance Abuse Treatment and Recovery* to address the needs of women with AOD abuse problems (Moore et al., 1995). This adapted curriculum is used widely in the AOD abuse treatment system in Massachusetts as well as nationally. Camp and Finkelstein (1997) reported that this intervention, one of CSAP's model/exemplary parenting programs, improved parenting as measured on objective scales and also enhanced parents' satisfaction and competency (Camp & Finkelstein, 1997; Moore & Finkelstein, 2001). As part of the WELL Project, IHR adapted this curriculum to include information on co-occurring disorders and trauma. Some sessions were rewritten, increasing the focus on skill-building and limiting the amount of self-exploration/self-disclosure, in order to reduce the risk of traumatic memories being triggered. This new program, entitled *Nurturing Families Affected by Substance Abuse, Mental Illness, and Trauma*, is designed to increase women's awareness of the impact of AOD abuse, mental illness, and trauma on themselves and their children and develop skills to promote healing in relationships with their children. The fourteen, 90-minute sessions consist of experiential exercises followed by participatory discussions on topics such as safety and protecting children, self-esteem, setting boundaries, children's feelings, and guiding behaviors. The group offers opportunities to address shame and guilt, self-acceptance, impact of trauma on women and children, children's developmental milestones, appropriate expectations, effective discipline strategies, and parenting techniques. This parenting intervention was offered at the three sites in both residential and outpatient settings. Groups were led by Parent-Child Specialists from IHR, co-facilitated by local site clinicians when available.

Peer-Led Mutual Help Groups

Women with co-occurring disorders and histories of trauma often report that existing self-help groups do not meet their needs. Some object to some of the 12-step language, especially references to powerlessness. Others find a bias against medication among members or do not feel it appropriate to discuss either mental illness or trauma in that forum. Therefore, a third intervention developed was a gender-specific mutual help model specifically for women with these three issues developed by consumers familiar with self-help. The Director of the Peer Educators Project at Vinfen and the Consumer Coordinator of the WELL Project worked together to develop a model called WELL Recovery. WELL Recovery meetings have a format similar to other self-help groups such as AA or Double Trouble, but do not include the twelve steps. Trained consumers facilitate the meetings in which participants share their strength, experience and hope around specific topics chosen by the group. The WELL Recovery manual, available from IHR, describes how to start and run a WELL Recovery group and contains lists of suggested topics and quotes to use in conjunction with the groups.

The Consumer Coordinator of the WELL Project recruited, trained, and supervised peer facilitators who led groups in the communities served by the three local sites. Peer facilitators were paid for their work by Vinfen under a contract from Massachusetts' Medicaid managed care vendor.

WELL Child Project

The WELL Child Project, one of four sites funded by SAMHSA as a Children's Sub-Study, was located at two of the WELL Project sites. This project, part of a cross-site, exploratory, pooled data study, provided clinical screening and assessment services, individualized resource coordination and advocacy, and a skill-building/trauma-informed group intervention to children ages 5-10 of mothers who were WELL Project participants and who agreed to their children's participation. Two staffpersons called Child Clinician Advocates (CCAs) worked with the children and their mothers with the goal of influencing positive outcomes in safety, self-care, relationships and identity. The WELL Child Project served 26 children at the two intervention sites and enrolled 21 at the comparison site.

CONCLUSION

What has been demonstrated by the WELL Project is the possibility of using a relational, collaborative model to bring about change at multiple levels of a service delivery system. Strategies such as bringing all stakeholders to the table, especially consumers, and then engaging in values clarification, providing cross-training, and creating a safe environment for dialogue are effective in preparing the ground for change. Working together, stakeholders can then create a model for service delivery that best meets the needs of all concerned.

The response of participating agencies as the WELL Project draws to a close provides some information about its impact. Executive Directors of all three agencies were unanimous in concluding that the resource coordination and advocacy services were enormously helpful to the women and agency staff, and they expressed a strong desire to find a funding source to continue these services. One Executive Director included resource coordination and advocacy services in a successful federal drug court grant application. All three Executive Directors were equally enthusiastic about *Seeking Safety* groups and plan to continue them after the project ends. The Director of a women's residential program at one site indicated she believed the trauma groups had an important impact on staff at her program, increasing their comfort in dealing with trauma symptoms such as self-harm and flashbacks. She is currently working on adapting *Seeking Safety* for use with adolescents, so that groups can be conducted in an adolescent residential program at her agency as well.

Members of the LLCs are also reluctant to see the WELL Project end. A member agency of one of the LLCs has offered to provide space, minutes and mailings so that the work can continue. In another community, the Regional Domestic Violence Council chose to absorb the LLC as a "Subcommittee on Integration" so the LLC work can continue.

The WELL Project has increased the awareness of administrators, providers and consumers of the benefits of trauma-informed, integrated services. Outcome data from the WCDV study will be useful in further fueling, directing, and disseminating efforts to make such services available to all women with co-occurring disorders and histories of violence.

REFERENCES

Beckman, L.J. & Amaro, H. (1986). Personal and social difficulties faced by women and men entering alcoholism treatment. *Journal of Studies on Alcohol, 47(2)*, 135-145.

Bollerud, K. (1990). A model for the treatment of trauma related syndromes among chemically dependent inpatient women. *Journal of Substance Abuse Treatment, 7*, 83-87.

Camp, J.M. & Finkelstein, N. (1997). Parenting training for women in residential substance abuse treatment: Results of a demonstration project. *Journal of Substance Abuse Treatment, 14(5)*, 411-422.

Covington, S.S. & Surrey, J. (2000). The relational model of women's psychological development: Implications for substance abuse. *Work in Progress* No. 91. Wellesley, MA: Stone Center Working Paper Series.

Cramer, M. (2001). *"Introduction," WELL Project Training Curriculum for Providers: Developing Integrated Services for Women with Substance Abuse, Mental Illness and Trauma.* Cambridge, MA: Institute for Health and Recovery.

Fedele, N.M. & Harrington, E. (1990). Women's groups: How connections heal. *Work in Progress* No. 47. Wellesley, MA: Stone Center Working Paper Series.

Finkelstein, N. (1994). Treatment issues for alcohol- and drug-dependent pregnant and parenting women. *Health and Social Work, 19(1),* 7-15.

Finkelstein, N. (1996). Using the relational model as a context for treating pregnant and parenting chemically dependent women. *Journal of Chemical Dependency Treatment, 6(1/2),* 23-44.

Finkelstein, N., Kennedy, C., Thomas, K., & Kearnes, M. (1997) *Gender-Specific Substance Abuse Treatment.* Alexandria, VA: National Women's Resource Center for the Prevention and Treatment of Alcohol, Tobacco, and Other Drug Abuse and Mental Illness.

Harris, M. (1994). Modifications in service delivery and clinical treatment for women diagnosed with severe mental illness who are survivors of sexual abuse trauma. *Journal of Mental Health Administration, 21(4),* 397-406.

Harris, M. & Fallot, R.D. (2001). *Using Trauma Theory to Design Service Systems.* San Francisco: Jossey-Bass.

Harvey, M.R. & Harney, P.A. (1997). Addressing the aftermath of interpersonal violence: The case for long term care. *Psychoanalytic Inquiry, 1997 Supplement,* 29-44.

Institute for Health and Recovery (2001). *WELL Project Training Curriculum for Providers: Developing Integrated Services for Women with Substance Abuse, Mental Illness and Trauma.* Cambridge, MA: Institute for Health and Recovery.

Jordan, J., Kaplan, A., Miller, J., Stiver, I., & Surry, J. (1991). *Women's Growth in Connection: Writings from the Stone Center.* New York: Guilford Press.

Lyons-Ruth, K. & Block, D. (1996). The disturbed caregiving system: Relations among childhood trauma, maternal caregiving, and infant affect and attachment. *Infant Mental Health Journal, 17,* 257-275.

Markoff, L.S. & Cawley, P.A. (1996). Retaining our clients and our sanity: A multi-systems model of case management. *Journal of Chemical Dependency Treatment, Special Issue-Chemical Dependency: Women at Risk, 6,* 45-65.

Miller, J.B. (2002). How change happens: Controlling images, mutuality and power. *Work in Progress* No. 96. Wellesley, MA: Stone Center Working Paper Series.

Minkoff, K. (2001). Developing standards of care for individuals with co-occurring psychiatric and substance use disorders. *Psychiatric Services, 52, No.5,* 597-599.

Moore, J., Buchan, B., Finkelstein, N., & Thomas, K. (1995). *Nurturing Program for Families in Substance Abuse Treatment and Recovery.* Park City, Utah: Family Development Resources, Inc.

Moore, J. & Finkelstein, N. (2001). Parenting services for families affected by substance abuse. *Child Welfare League of America, LXXX,* 221-238.

Mulford, H.A. (1977). Women and men problem drinkers: Sex differences in patients served by Iowa's community alcoholism center. *Journal of Studies on Alcohol, 38,* 1624-1639.

Najavits, L. (2002). *Seeking Safety: A Treatment Manual for PTSD and Substance Abuse.* New York, NY: Guildford Press.

Najavits, L.M., Gastfriend, D.R., Barber, J.P., Reif, S., Muenz, L.R., Blaine, J., Frank, A., Crists-Christoph, P., Thase, M., & Weiss, R.D. (1998). Cocaine dependence with and without posttraumatic stress disorder among subjects in the NIDA Collaborative Cocaine Treatment Study. *American Journal of Psychiatry, 155,* 214-219.

Seval-Brooks, C. & Fitzgerald-Rice, K. (1997). *Families in Recovery Coming Full Circle.* Baltimore, MD: Brooks Publishing Co.

Van Bremen, J.R. & Chasnoff, I.J. (1994). Policy issues for integrating parenting interventions and addiction treatment for women. *Topics in Early Childhood Special Education, 14,* 254-274.

A Model for Changing Alcohol and Other Drug, Mental Health, and Trauma Services Practice: PROTOTYPES Systems Change Center

Vivian B. Brown, PhD
Elke Rechberger, PhD
Paula Bjelajac

SUMMARY. Despite the high rates of trauma in the lives of women with alcohol and other drug abuse, and mental health disorders, little is known about best practices for this population. PROTOTYPES, Centers for Innovation in Health, Mental Health, and Social Services only focused on demonstrating the effectiveness of a new integrated model of treatment for women with co-occurring disorders and trauma and their children, as well as on systems integration and systems change. This paper describes the three levels of integration the PROTOTYPES' Systems Change Center implemented during the five-year project: services integration, systems integration, and consumer/survivor/recovering integration. *[Article copies available for a fee from The Haworth Document Delivery Service: 1-800-HAWORTH. E-mail address: <docdelivery@haworthpress.*

Vivian B. Brown, Elke Rechberger, and Paula Bjelajac are affiliated with PROTOTYPES.

The authors wish to thank Sylvia DeGraff for her assistance and patience in the presentation of this manuscript.

[Haworth co-indexing entry note]: "A Model for Changing Alcohol and Other Drug, Mental Health, and Trauma Services Practice: PROTOTYPES Systems Change Center." Brown, Vivian B., Elke Rechberger, and Paula Bjelajac. Co-published simultaneously in *Alcoholism Treatment Quarterly* (The Haworth Press, Inc.) Vol. 22, No. 3/4, 2004, pp. 81-94; and: *Responding to Physical and Sexual Abuse in Women with Alcohol and Other Drug and Mental Disorders: Program Building* (ed: Bonita M. Veysey, and Colleen Clark) The Haworth Press, Inc., 2004, pp. 81-94. Single or multiple copies of this article are available for a fee from The Haworth Document Delivery Service [1-800-HAWORTH, 9:00 a.m. - 5:00 p.m. (EST). E-mail address: docdelivery@haworthpress.com].

com> Website: <http://www.HaworthPress.com> © 2004 by The Haworth Press, Inc. All rights reserved.]

KEYWORDS. Alcoholism, drug abuse, women, physical abuse, sexual abuse, integration

INTRODUCTION

Professionals working with individuals diagnosed with co-occurring disorders face challenging dilemmas about how to provide the best treatment to address more than one condition. Despite the high rates of trauma in the lives of women with alcohol and other drug (AOD) abuse and mental health disorders, little is known about best practices for this population. Women-sensitive programs have been described over the past decades (Reed, 1987; Finkelstein, 1993; Brown, 2000). These programs are based on women's unique needs; e.g., histories of childhood and adulthood sexual and physical abuse necessitating safe and nurturing environments for treatment. Ideally, they are structured so that mothers do not have to be separated from their children and that their children are provided with treatment services. However, trauma-informed, gender-specific treatments needed to be studied for women with co-occurring disorders.

PROTOTYPES, Centers for Innovation in Health, Mental Health and Social Services, a private, nonprofit, community-based organization, was founded in 1986 to serve disenfranchised and underserved communities of Los Angeles County in California. With 25 locations in Southern California, the agency serves over 10,000 women and children, and family members each year through the provision of AOD treatment, HIV/AIDS prevention and care, mental health treatment, and trauma services. Its focus on women and children is in direct response to inadequate and fragmented systems of care for women and women with children. In addition to its service programs, PROTOTYPES also has major training, research, and dissemination programs to bring research to practice.

Systems change is part of PROTOTYPES' mission. Systems change means developing or significantly improving programs that integrate mental health, AOD, trauma, health and HIV/AIDS. This is accomplished by demonstrating effectiveness of these integrated programs for women with multiple vulnerabilities, providing training and technical assistance to assist communities and providers to implement evidence-based interventions, convening new networks of policy makers, practitioners, researchers, and consumers to define new strategies, and fostering new policies on key issues. The PROTOTYPES Systems Change Center focuses on systems integration and change, as well as on demonstrating the effectiveness of a new model of treatment for women with co-occurring disorders and traumas.

WOMEN WITH CO-OCCURRING DISORDERS AND TRAUMA PROJECT

Issues of services integration and systems change within the context of welfare reform were discussed from the beginning of the project in 1998. The coming of welfare reform to California offered some unusual opportunities for integrating services to women welfare clients needing assistance with problems of AOD problems, mental illness and domestic violence. The pioneering efforts of the L.A. County Department of Public Social Services in this realm provided direct experience with integrated services for a large number of women with multiple vulnerabilities. In addition, the CalWORKS program also allowed for the expansion of mental health services to welfare recipients who may not be severely mentally ill, but have other DSM-IV diagnoses.

Utilizing welfare reform as a catalyst for change also allowed PROTOTYPES to demonstrate a number of models of outreach and service delivery, such as registration of women for CalWORKS at the treatment site (in addition to CalWORKS offices), co-location of staff, cross-training, and improved assessments.

Systems Integration

PROTOTYPES commitment to systems integration is multidimensional. The guiding philosophy underlying systems integration is that change must occur at both the macro and the micro level. Systems change must happen at the top levels of administration, where policies are created, but systems change also needs to occur at the most basic level, with the front-line staff who serve clients, and incorporating input from the client peer community of consumer/survivor/recovering persons. Systems integration also must include collateral systems such as criminal justice, welfare, and education. Policy and service systems, from state and county administrators, to judges, to schools, and all other provider agencies that interact with a particular client, work together to provide a more seamless service delivery, and better outcomes for clients.

As can been seen in Figure 1, PROTOTYPES designed a systems change effort beginning with the innermost circle, the PROTOTYPES Women's Center Programs. The next circle represents the 25 PROTOTYPES sites that were the next level of technology transfer. After the PROTOTYPES expanded system, there is the Service Planning Area (SPA 3) that involves over 50 agencies providing services. The next level involves the entire Los Angeles County Systems, including mental health, AOD, TANF, health and HIV/AIDS. The last level is the State Systems.

FIGURE 1. Levels of Systems Change

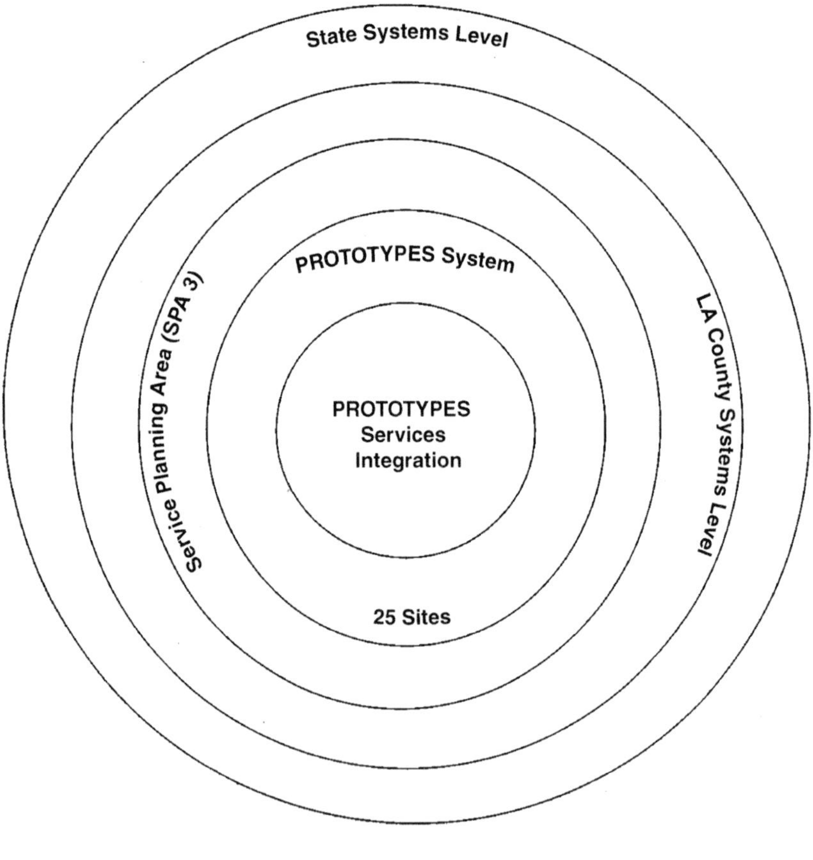

PROTOTYPES participation in systems integration is manifested at all levels of administrative and policy systems (see Table 1). PROTOTYPES staff participate on the national level by serving on multiple advisory committees on co-occurring disorders; at the state level, by providing leadership on the California Co-Occurring Disorders Task Force and serving on the Women's Mental Health Council; at the County level, by serving as a member of the Narcotics and Dangerous Drugs Commission (NDDC), and the HIV/AIDS Commission. At the local level, PROTOTYPES not only participates in existing system roles, but has also created new planning bodies and committees to help aid systems integration in the community. The creation of the *Local Experts Group* (LEG) in 1997 provided an opportunity for policy makers, researchers, providers, and consumer/survivor/recovering persons to meet and discuss the need for system integration and provide assistance to help make those changes occur. Key participants in the LEG include both the previous and the current Directors of the Los Angeles County Department of Mental Health, as well as the previous and current Directors of the Los Angeles County Alcohol and Drug Program Administration, and the Director of the Los Angeles County Department of Public and Social Services. Los Angeles County has separate service systems for mental health, AOD problems, domestic violence, and HIV/AIDS, among others, to treat the 10 million constituents under their care. The ability of the *Local Experts Group* to bring together the key public policy makers, service providers, and consumers in one organizational body has been a primary mechanism to effect change within the larger service systems.

At the local service provider level, PROTOTYPES provided leadership in the development of the *Dual Diagnosis Staff Development Committee* in 1999 to facilitate bringing all treatment staff to optimal levels of best practice in outreach, screening and assessment, treatment, and continuing care and support services for clients. Key participants in this organization include mid-level administrative staff, service area coordinators, program directors, and front-line staff from the Los Angeles County Department of Mental Health, Los Angeles County Department of Alcohol and Drug Program Administration, and Los Angeles County Department of Education.

Out of this body, a five-year Staff Development Plan was developed, including: (a) Executive Briefings on current research, protocol, and policy for the administrative staff from all the various local governing agencies; (b) Training of Trainers, so all service area coordinators are able to train local staff on best practices; (c) an annual *Co-Occurring*

TABLE 1

Macro Level	Micro Level
DPSS/DMH/ADPA	LA Partners
NDDC	SAAC-III
CASCs	Westside Mental Health
Local Experts Group (LEG)	SPA 3 Meetings
County Staff Development Committee	Schools
State Co-Occurring Disorders Task Force	Judges
	Consumer Advisory Group/Peer Advocates

Disorders Across the Lifespan conference, which disseminates information on latest research and treatment developments, as well as provide opportunities for interagency collaborations; and (d) Cross-Training and Technical Assistance for local provider agencies.

PROTOTYPES has been involved in other system integration efforts, including the planning and implementation of one of eight Community Service Assessment Centers (CASC) in 2000 by the Los Angeles County Alcohol and Drug Program Administration. The CASCs act as central intake and assessment centers for AOD, mental health, trauma, and HIV agencies. The populations served by the CASCs include: CalWORKS (TANF), Proposition 36, General Relief clients, and other Community clients. Although the primary function of the CASCs is to provide assessments of clients and place them all into appropriate treatment services, a number of concomitant system integration efforts have occurred as a result of their existence in the community.

Knowledge dissemination efforts have included trainings for front-line staff, and technical assistance to treatment programs. These efforts provided opportunities for community organization and interagency collaborations, changing how treatment is provided, providing feedback to the larger governing bodies about specific system change needs. One recent manifestation of such a change was the recommendation of 8 additional questions on trauma in the initial assessment measure.

Services Integration

At PROTOTYPES Women's Center, the integrated model is distinguished by the fact that service integration is achieved by providing all services on-site. PROTOTYPES Women's Center services are based on the following guidelines: (a) women are seen in their multiple roles as women, as drug users, as mothers, as relationship partners, as members of extended families, and as at risk for multiple problems; (b) the quality of the residential treatment environment must reinforce the message that the women and children require and deserve a warm, nurturing, and safe environment; (c) women in staff positions, including management of the agency are role models and send an important message to clients about women's value and abilities; (d) treatment emphasizes empowerment of the women, enhances her ability to identify and express her needs, and encourages her to determine the direction that treatment, as well as her life will take; and (e) treatment services need to integrate the most up-to-date information and promising practices.

PROTOTYPES had previously demonstrated that its residential treatment model for women and children was effective (Brown, Huba & Melchior, 1998). PROTOTYPES Women's Center is a modified therapeutic community (Sacks et al., 1997; Brown et al., 1996). To enhance the level of service integration, it was important to choose a powerful, evidence-based intervention integrating AOD, mental health, and trauma that could be embedded into the present model. Effective psychosocial treatments are important for individuals for whom early abstinence may be associated with a worsening of psychiatric symptoms, such as women with PTSD who may experience anxiety when they cease alcohol use (Petrakis et al., 2002).

The central role of trauma in the lives of vulnerable women is a fundamental component of this model, and of the PROTOTYPES approach to integrated services. Increasingly, sexual and physical violence is seen as an underlying factor both creating and aggravating other problems such as AOD abuse, mental illness, and HIV/AIDS. While integrated approaches need to provide a response to all of a woman's complex needs, putting trauma "up front" in both a practical and philosophical sense responds to current science about the origins of multiple vulnerability, and to the voice of C/S/R representatives about the importance of empowering women to address the issues of trauma.

To develop an enhanced intervention, PROTOTYPES staff investigated a number of trauma-specific group curricula, including TREM (Harris, 1998), *Seeking Safety* (Najavits, 2001), *Helping Women Recover* (Covington, 1999), and EMDR (Shapiro, 1996). PROTOTYPES arranged full-day training visits by Dr. Maxine Harris and Dr. Lisa Najavits, and the Principal Investigator of PROTOTYPES took EMDR training. A clinical group consisting of Dr. Brown and other highly experienced clinicians held a day-long retreat to compare the 4 models.

The outcome was the choice of *Seeking Safety*. The strengths identified were: (a) sequence flexibility, (b) strong AOD/recovery perspective, (c) coverage of HIV, (d) personal sensitivity of Dr. Najavits to the population, (e) impressive conceptual bases and research evidence for *Seeking Safety*, (f) formalized curriculum in a manual, and (g) compatibility with what PROTOTYPES was already doing with respect to holding groups for trauma survivors.

The *Seeking Safety* curriculum was open to changing sequence of sessions and changing number of sessions devoted to a topic to reflect emphasis on particular issues. On the basis of feedback after a pilot test of the curriculum, the curriculum was extended to 31 sessions by having 2 sessions for certain topics. C/S/R feedback was pivotal in the decision to choose *Seeking Safety*, and in the modifications of sequence and number of sessions.

In *Seeking Safety*, the theme of safety wraps around everything, not just in response to PTSD symptoms but also, e.g., discussing HIV in a safety framework. The session on "grounding" teaches a tool to use when trauma comes up, so that the woman is not in danger of being flooded. It was also decided that the groups would be co-led by C/S/Rs, and mental health professionals.

Trauma-informed services address the following women-sensitive needs: biological/physical, psychosocial, support service, informational and educational, vocational, parenting, and reparenting. Activities for physical/health needs include on-site health screening, child immunizations, prenatal groups, and HIV/AIDS groups. Activities for meeting psychosocial needs include specialized treatment groups that focus on specific trauma (e.g., sexual and physical abuse, domestic violence, etc.), unresolved grief and loss issues, anger management and positive use of anger, life skills building, individual counseling, family counseling, and relapse prevention. Informational and educational activities include physical effects of alcohol and other drug use, nutrition, women's health issues, eating disorders, HIV/AIDS risk reduction, and women's issues in recovery. Parenting activities include parenting skills training, "Mommy and Me" classes, a pregnancy support group, mother-child outings, and the Parenting Center. In addition, there are services for mental health and AOD treatment.

The PROTOTYPES Women's Center provides a residential program lasting from 12 to 18 months duration. This long-term focus allows for a number of advantages for the women: (1) women who are pregnant can enter early in their pregnancy and stay beyond the birth in order to learn parenting skills; (2) women who have lost custody but wish to work toward reuniting with their children have sufficient treatment time to do so; and (3) women with multiple vulnerabilities, including high psychological distress, have sufficient time to show reduced impairment. The high incidence of depression, low self-esteem and histories of sexual and physical abuse necessitates sufficient time and pacing in order to not overwhelm or flood the women with anxiety and feelings of helplessness.

PROTOTYPES serves a population representative of the racial-ethnic make-up of the Los Angeles area: white/Caucasians (32%), black/African Americans (33%), Hispanic/Latinas (32%), Asian/Pacific Islander (2%), and American Indian (1%).

For PROTOTYPES, services integration involves bringing together, in one organizational unit, a range of services that are delivered in a unified way by one treatment team for the purpose of improved outcomes for the consumers. In the PROTOTYPES Pomona facility, medical staff, mental health staff, AOD staff, vocational training staff, and children's staff are all brought together in teams to plan treatment, provide treatment services, and plan community re-entry. As part of these teams, it is important to note that 50% of the staff are/have been consumers.

C/S/R Integration

Women identified as victims of violence can suffer for many years with symptoms of undiagnosed posttraumatic stress disorder (PTSD) and major depression, as well as have symptoms of hearing voices and dissociation. These symptoms can be initiated by the violence they have experienced (i.e., domestic violence, incest, rape, physical violence, witnessing an act of violence). Alcohol and/or other drugs are abused to eliminate these symptoms and make one "feel better." When victims of violence turn to substances they find themselves in very unsafe situations, which may lead to further victimization, trigger their PTSD, continue retraumatization, and becoming trapped in a downward spiral.

Women who fall into this trap can remain stuck for many years feeling there is no exit. For the lucky few who find treatment, some never remember how they got to the treatment facility. They may not have been sober or experiencing symptoms from their mental illness. Today, many clients have barriers to sobriety and stopping the downward spiral. Women present with more than one need or problem (i.e., AOD, mental illness, trauma, medical issues–hepatitis C, HIV/AIDS). If we want treatment to be a success for our clients, then all of these issues need to be addressed. The last element in a trauma-informed model is Consumer/Survivor/Recovery Integration.

Alcoholics Anonymous (AA) works because it is one alcoholic talking to another. Often, alcoholics enter into the program of AA having reached the depths of personal misery. By listening to others who have been in the program for some time, they begin to relate to the personal stories and their desire to want what the others have grows. They keep coming back, beginning the process of recovery.

Unfortunately, AA cannot reach all groups of individuals. For those who are victims of violent crimes, their voices are often never heard. Victims live in a world of fear, denial, helplessness, and hopelessness. The recovery process begins for the victims of violence when they are given the opportunity to listen to others who have moved from victim to survivor. The same is true for those who suffer from a mental illness. The healing process begins when one trauma survivor talks to another, one mentally ill person talks to another, one alcoholic/addict talks to another.

Once the CSR has found her/his voice, they must be involved in establishing standards of care that will be used to shape integrated systems of the future (Brown, 1997). It is not enough for a CSR to only bond with another alcoholic. If that person is unaware of the complexities for those of multiple vulnerabilities, it could be harmful to the newcomer. For a sponsor who knows nothing about PTSD, or schizophrenia, she may be suggesting to her sponsee to stop taking her psychotropic medications because she is not really "clean." If this advice is followed, this could be a dangerous situation for the newcomer, as she becomes symptomatic with her schizophrenia once again, possibly leading her back to using substances, and/or hospitalization.

As providers of services begin to integrate the treatment needs of multiple vulnerabilities, they must include CSRs at every level of their agency. Consumers who have experienced the effects of trauma, AOD abuse, and mental illness need to be heard. In an empowerment model the Consumer/Survivor/Recovering person is the expert.

"PROTOTYPES is a transformational, woman-oriented culture that is 'fluid, it is a place where ideas can percolate, where ambiguity is tolerated, and all staff members are important.' This culture fosters role modeling for consumer staff and promotes belief in their abilities" (Brown & Worth, 2002 pg. 36). "I found out early on that if I brought an idea to the CEO, I must be ready to follow through. If she encouraged me to bring my ideas to fruition it meant next week, not next year" (Paula Bjelajac, personal communication). "This level of accountability promotes staff members respecting themselves, helps raise their self-esteem and gives incentive to keep on going. The level of expectation of competence gives staff a lot of responsibility but it also gives them more freedom to exercise that responsibility working alone and as part of a team" (Brown & Worth, 2002 pg. 37).

The experience of PROTOTYPES consumer staff indicates that a number of benefits arise for the consumer. Significant benefits may include: (a) having the opportunity to give back, "We can only keep what we have by giving it away" (AA); (b) being respected for who they are, and for their life experiences; (c) earning a salary; (d) continuing their education, women are encouraged to go back to school, have a career, and move ahead; (e) rebuilding self-esteem; (f) being empowered; (g) learning to overcome victimization, to trust, possibly for the first time in their lives; (h) learning new skills; (i) learning to become open minded, non-judgmental, "to see beyond the labels applied to many consumers" (Brown & Worth, 2002); (j) teaching others–by disclosing, others learn from us; (k) learning to set boundaries; and (l) decreasing isolation.

The benefits of integrating consumer/survivor/recovery persons into all levels of system and service and evaluation efforts range from improving the quality of services and performance improvement to increasing overall organizational efficacy (McCabe & Unzicker, 1995; Campbell, 1993; Fisher, 1994; Deegan, 1995).

Some barriers to integration of the CSR may include: (a) salary and benefits–issues of pay vs. disability payments; fear of getting off disability; (b) boundary issues; transference/countertransference issues; (c) confidentiality issues; need for ongoing training on confidentiality regulations; (d) training and supervision; need for adequate orientation period; need for training in work ethic; (e) relapse alcohol and mental illness issues; need for support/recovery system and flexibility in schedules and workload; (f) retraumatization; agency should be trauma informed; (g) organizational/cultural issues; support for new opportunities and roles for consumer staff require systems to redefine their missions and cultures (Brown & Worth, 2002).

Within the 25 PROTOTYPES agencies, at least 50% of the staff members are CSRs. From directors to AOD counselors, CSRs fit into all levels. Depending on the facility, recruiting consumer staff whose experience, age, ethnicity, etc., are similar to the client population is certainly a criterion. A special recruitment criterion for specific consumer staff working with clients with multiple vulnerabilities was developed.

Recruitment criteria for consumer staff to work with clients with co-occurring disorders, and survivors of trauma should include (taken from the recruiting manual):

- Experience with mental illness, or mental illness and alcoholism and recovery
- A personal history of experiencing trauma
- A personal support system in place (self-help, faith-based support, etc.)
- A safety plan and resources in place in case of a crisis

CSRs are employed at every level throughout the PROTOTYPES agency. Examples of various positions for CSRs include: Deputy Director of PROTOTYPES comprehensive treatment program, Case Manager, Substance Abuse Counselor, Group Facilitator for co-occurring disorders, Seeking Safety co-facilitator, along with a mental health professional, Members of the Staff Development Dual Disorders Committee, Members of the Local Experts Group, Presenter at various conferences and colleges, Data Coordinator, Trainer, HIV Counselors, Peer Support, Intake workers, Outreach workers, Research Assistants.

LESSONS LEARNED

Implications for future research and systems change are three-fold: this project highlights increased awareness of trauma as a critical factor in women's lives that needs to be addressed, helps providers recognize the need to rethink diagnostic criteria to one that is more broadly inclusive than previously existed, and demonstrates a need to incorporate trauma as a systems integration issue.

In terms of increasing awareness, educating providers about the issue of trauma helps them comprehend the concept of co-occurring disorders more readily. When talking about the co-occurring disorders of alcoholism/other drug abuse and mental illness, it is often difficult for individuals to grasp how the two disorders may be interwoven with each other. Demonstrating that early, unresolved trauma issues may have been the precursor to the development of either or both substance use and mental health disorders in a woman's life helps provide a link to understanding how all three issues are intermingled in etiology and symptomatology. Such awareness undergirds the premise that frequently the clients we provide services for have more than one disorder that needs clinical intervention, which may also be best provided for in an integrated treatment model.

Rethinking diagnostic criteria so that co-occurring disorders are more broadly defined is also a necessary change. Historically, co-occurring disorders in terms of mental health was defined only by those clients suffering from severe and persistent mental illness (e.g., schizophrenia). Understanding the etiology of trauma also helps focus the discussion of co-occurring disorders to include those women who may have Posttraumatic Stress Disorder as a co-occurring mental health issue (or complex trauma issues that do not meet *DSM-IV* criteria for PTSD), along with more severe AOD issues.

Finally, it is important to recognize that trauma is not only at the intersection of AOD problems and mental illness, but also is the critical juncture point for which welfare, criminal justice, homelessness, and health services interact. Awareness that all these systems intersect around the co-occurring issue of trauma can educate all providers to become more trauma-sensitive, and provide services which are trauma-informed.

REFERENCES

Brown, V.B., Huba, G.J., & Melchior, L. (1995). Level of burden: women with more than one co-occurring disorder. *Journal of Psychoactive Drugs*, 27 (4), 339-346.

Brown, V.B., Sanchez, S., Zweben, J.E., & Aly, J. (1996). Challenges in moving from a traditional therapeutic community to a women and children's therapeutic community model. *Journal of Psychoactive Drugs*, 28 (1), 39-46.

Brown, V.B., & Worth, D. (2002). *Recruiting, training and maintaining consumer staff: strategies used and lessons learned.* PROTOTYPES Systems Change Center.

Campbell, J., Ralph, R., & Glover, R. (1993). From lab rat to researcher: The history, models, and policy implications of consumer/survivor involvement in research. proceedings: Fourth annual national conference on state mental health agency services research and program evaluation. NASMHPD, Alexandria, VA, 138-157.

Covington, S. (1999). *Helping women recover: a program for treating substance abuse.* San Francisco, CA: Jossey-Bass.

Deegan, P.E. (1995). Recovery as a journey of the heart. Presented at recovery from psychiatric disability: implication for the training of mental health professionals, Massachusetts State House, May 10.

Finkelstein, N. (1993). Treatment programming for alcohol and drug dependent pregnant women. *International Journal of Addictions*, 28 (13).

Fisher, D. (1994). A new vision of healing as constructed by people with psychiatric disabilities working as mental health providers. *Psychosocial Rehabilitation Journal*, 17 (3), 67-81.

Harris, M. (1998). *Trauma recovery and empowerment.* New York: The Free Press.

McCabe, S. & Unzicker, R.E., (1995). Changing roles of consumer/survivors in mature mental health systems. *New Directions for Mental Health Services* 66 (summer), 61-73. Jossey-Bass Publishers.

Najavits, L.M. (2002). *Seeking safety: a treatment manual for PTSD and substance abuse.* New York: Guilford Press.

Petrakis, I.L., Gonzalez, G., Rosenbeck, R., & Krystal, J.H. (2002). Comorbidity of alcoholism and psychiatric disorders: an overview. *Alcohol Research & Health,* 26 (No. 2), 81-89.

Reed, B.G. (1985). Drug misuse and dependency in women: the meaning and implications of being considered a special population or minority group. *International Journal of Addictions,* 20, 13-62.

Sacks, S., DeLeon, G., Bernhardt, A.I., & Sacks, J.Y. (1997). A modified therapeutic community for homeless mentally ill chemical abusers. In G. DeLeon (Ed.) *Community as method: therapeutic communities for special populations and special settings.* Westport, CT: Greenwood Publishing Group, 19-37.

Shapiro, F. (1996). Eye movement desensitization and reprocessing: basic principles, protocols and procedures.

Boston Consortium of Services for Families in Recovery: A Trauma-Informed Intervention Model for Women's Alcohol and Drug Addiction Treatment

Hortensia Amaro, PhD
Sarah McGraw, PhD
Mary Jo Larson, PhD
Luz Lopez, MSW, MPH
Rita Nieves, RN, MPH
Brenda Marshall

Hortensia Amaro is affiliated with the Institute on Urban Health Research, Northeastern University. Sarah McGraw and Mary Jo Larson are affiliated with the New England Research Institutes. Luz Lopez, Rita Nieves, and Brenda Marshall are affiliated with Boston Public Health Commission.

The authors would like to recognize the contributions of the members of the Boston Consortium of Services for Families in Recovery, New England Research Institutes, and women in recovery whose participation and input were essential in the development and implementation of the intervention and evaluation. They would also like to thank the Project Officers, Susan Salasin and Kana Enamoto, who provided guidance and support to the Consortium team during the implementation process. The work reported in this paper was supported by the Substance Abuse and Mental Health Services Administration, Grant Number: TI11397.

[Haworth co-indexing entry note]: "Boston Consortium of Services for Families in Recovery: A Trauma-Informed Intervention Model for Women's Alcohol and Drug Addiction Treatment." Amaro, Hortensia et al. Co-published simultaneously in *Alcoholism Treatment Quarterly* (The Haworth Press, Inc.) Vol. 22, No. 3/4, 2004, pp. 95-119; and: *Responding to Physical and Sexual Abuse in Women with Alcohol and Other Drug and Mental Disorders: Program Building* (ed: Bonita M. Veysey, and Colleen Clark) The Haworth Press, Inc., 2004, pp. 95-119. Single or multiple copies of this article are available for a fee from The Haworth Document Delivery Service [1-800-HAWORTH, 9:00 a.m. - 5:00 p.m. (EST). E-mail address: docdelivery@haworthpress.com].

SUMMARY. Through collaboration among the service agencies collectively known as the Boston Consortium of Services for Families in Recovery, the Boston Public Health Commission implemented an integrated model of trauma-informed services that is culturally and linguistically appropriate to its service population of primarily poor urban Latina and African American women. The enhanced intervention was implemented in five Consortium-affiliated alcohol and drug addiction treatment programs providing outpatient, residential, and methadone services. Programs adopted trauma-informed service system enhancements and offered study participants a package of trauma-specific and trauma-informed clinical services. The assessment and consensus-building processes, enhanced model components, implementation process, challenges and lessons learned are described. *[Article copies available for a fee from The Haworth Document Delivery Service: 1-800-HAWORTH. E-mail address: <docdelivery@haworthpress.com> Website: <http://www.HaworthPress.com> © 2004 by The Haworth Press, Inc. All rights reserved.]*

KEYWORDS. Trauma services, alcohol and drug addiction treatment, mental health services, African American women, Latina women, service integration

INTRODUCTION

The Boston Consortium of Services for Families in Recovery (the Consortium), under the Boston Public Health Commission (BPHC), formed a partnership of various programs and stakeholders to develop integrated services for women with co-occurring alcohol and drug abuse addiction, mental health and trauma histories. Prior to implementation of the intervention, the BPHC and affiliated programs within the Consortium had a long history of providing alcohol and drug addiction treatment including methadone and drug-free outpatient and residential modalities. Clinicians reported that a significant proportion of women clients had mental disorders and/or a history of trauma. Yet, as in many alcohol and drug addiction treatment programs (Grella, 1996), there was no systematic or formal assessment process of co-occurring disorders; staff lacked training in trauma treatment, and coordination of services across systems of care was informal. Many clinicians and consumers felt the result was a disjointed system of care with little connection between alcohol and drug addiction, trauma, and mental health treatment.

Service and system integration approaches were developed in two phases. Phase 1, which lasted two years, focused on an assessment and planning process during which partnerships were solidified and intervention approaches were developed. Phase 2 involved the implementation of the interventions and evaluation of the enhanced model. Although the overarching goal of systems integration remained constant, the Consortium evolved in its structure, focus, and specific strategies during the formative Phase 1 period.

This paper describes developments during both phases including intervention implementation and challenges faced by the Consortium in enhancing its service model to provide integrated services. Also described are the initial context of the system of care, evolution of the integrated service program, target population, program services, and lessons learned through the development and implementation process.

LITERATURE REVIEW

Despite the proliferation of studies on violence against women during the past twenty years (Gelles & Conte, 1990; Browne & Bassuk, 1997), limited research is available on the experience of violence among Latina and African American women (Amaro et al., 1999; Senturia et al., 2000). Furthermore, although there is general agreement about the profound negative impact of interpersonal violence on women's substance use and mental health (Browne, 1991, 1993; Boyd, 1993; Brown, Huba & Melchior, 1995; Caetano et al., 2000; Fullilove et al., 1993; Goodman et al., 1997; Kilpatrick et al., 1997; Liebshutz, Mulvey & Samet, 1997; McCauley et al., 1997; Najavits, Weiss & Shaw, 1997; Polusny & Follette, 1995), little is known about effective interventions. Even less is known about the efficacy of trauma interventions among Latina and African American women (Chalk & King, 1998).

There is a growing awareness that ethnicity and culture are important factors in understanding the ways women respond to violence and the barriers they may face in seeking help (Dutton, Orloff & Aguilar Hass, 2000; Senturia et al., 2000). Latinos and African Americans now comprise 25.4 percent of the U.S. population (U.S. Bureau of the Census, 2002). Due to their disproportionately high rates of poverty (U.S. Bureau of the Census, 2002), Latinos and African Americans are more likely to rely on publicly funded alcohol and other drug (AOD) treatment programs. The consequences of alcohol and drug addiction such as HIV infection and incarceration have a disproportionate impact on these populations (Sentencing Project, 2003; Beck, Karlberg & Harrison, 2002; CDC, 2001). Acculturation is associated with increased risk of substance use among Latinas (Amaro et al., 1990). These combined characteristics place these women at risk for interpersonal violence, mental illness, and AOD problems. Limited access to culturally and linguistically appropriate AOD and other services to help women stay safe may mean that women of color, especially those with dual diagnoses of mental health and substance use disorders, are also more likely to fall through the cracks of our current system of care.

Even integrated treatment models may not be perceived as valuable by women from racial and ethnic minority groups or they may be ineffective if they do not appeal to cultural values or address specific barriers faced by target women. For example, culturally determined gender roles, strong ties to the family, and fear of telling outsiders about abuse and stigma related to mental illness may promote denial of abuse among Latina and African American women (Perilla, Bakeman & Norris, 1994; Senturia et al., 2000; West et al., 1998).

Furthermore, fewer economic resources and the resulting family stress (West, 1998; Jasinski, 1996; Kaufman Kantor, Jasinski & Aldarondo, 1994) place women of color at risk. Interpersonal violence occurs in a cultural context, and factors such as degree of acculturation (Eberstein & Frisbie, 1976; Sorenson & Telles, 1991; Kaufman Kantor et al., 1994; Jasinski, 1996; Okamura, Heras & Wong-Kerber, 1995), expectations about gender roles and power in relationships and normative values about gender roles may contribute to increased risk among some cultural/ethnic groups (Amaro et al., 2001; Amaro & Raj, 2000; Amaro & Hardy Fanta, 1995; Amaro et al., 1999; Fullilove et al., 1990; Kaufman Kantor et al., 1994; Marin et al., 1997; Perilla, Bakeman & Norris, 1994; Wingood & DiClemente, 2000). Thus, successful interventions must address cultural as well gender factors related to social norms about trauma and mental illness.

BOSTON CONSORTIUM TARGET POPULATION

Recruited into the intervention were adult women (N = 181) who met the following criteria: current alcohol and/or drug abuse disorders, history of physical or sexual abuse, diagnosed mental disorder in the previous five years, and at least two prior encounters with the mental health or addictions treatment systems. All participants were receiving alcohol and/or drug addiction treatment (residential: 37%; outpatient: 30.4%; methadone: 32.6%) at one of five Consortium-affiliated agencies. The majority of women self-identified as non-Hispanic African American/Black (38.8%) or Hispanic/Latina[1] (31.5%–primarily of Puerto Rican descent), whereas a minority identified as non-Hispanic White (26.5%) and non-Hispanic Other Race (3.3%). In addition, 13% were Spanish monolingual and were interviewed in Spanish; 94.5% had children; and 58% of the mothers currently had custody of children under the age of 18 years. Less than one-half were currently married (13%) or were in a relationship with a significant other or sexual partner (26%). The mean age of women in the intervention was 35.3 years (SD = 7.5). Nearly half (42%) had not completed high school or a general equivalence diploma and very few were employed part- or full-time (6%).

Race/Ethnic Differences

Table 1 presents these sample characteristics by race/ethnic group. [Note, seven women who self-identified with multiple racial groups or as non-Hispanic Other Race are not reported separately in the table but are included in the total.] In conducting race/ethnic comparisons, Chi-Square analyses were used for categorical variables, and t-test and analysis of variance test (ANOVA) were used for continuous variables. The association of race/ethnicity with type of treatment reflects the participation of one residential program that targets Latina women, and two residential programs that target African American women.

The groups had statistically significant differences in education and age. Latina women had lower educational attainment and were younger. Statistically significant differences by race/ethnicity were found on some indicators of mental health problems. African American women reported fewer mental health symptoms on the Brief Symptom Inventory (Derogatis & Melisaratos, 1983) than other racial/ethnic groups. Thus, they had lower global severity index scores and a smaller proportion exceeded the 'caseness' criterion score. There was a notable difference across race/ethnicity in the proportion receiving any psychotropic medication with the highest rate among Latina women and lowest rate among African American women. The groups did not differ statistically on the proportion reporting childhood or current traumatic events. A trend ($p < .06$) in the data suggests that African American women had lower average scores on trauma symptoms on the Post-traumatic Stress Diagnostic Scale (Foa et al., 1993) and were more likely to feel very or

TABLE 1. Race/Ethnicity Comparisons on Baseline Characteristics Among Intervention Participants

Characteristics	Black/African American	Latina	White	Total[e]	P value
Total N	68	57	49	181	
			Percent		P value
Modality					
Residential	36.8	47.4	22.5	37.0	.0007
Outpatient	33.8	36.8	22.5	30.4	
Methadone	29.4	15.8	55.1	32.6	
Ever had children	94.1	96.5	93.7	95.0	NS
Currently have custody of children < age 18[b]	63.6	48.1	59.5	57.9	NS
Education					
Less than high school	32.3	59.7	38.8	42.0	.0183
High school graduate	48.5	35.1	42.9	43.1	
Some college or more	19.1	5.3	18.4	14.9	
Employment					
Some employment	10.3	1.7	6.1	6.1	NS
Unemployed	30.9	19.3	18.4	24.3	
Disabled	25.0	45.6	40.8	34.8	
In tx, homemaker, student	33.8	33.3	34.7	34.8	
Married or with partner	35.3	40.3	43.7	38.9	NS
BSI probable case[c]	80.9	94.7	95.9	88.4	.0096
Prescribed psychiatric meds in past 3 months	39.7	72.2	56.5	54.9	.0016
Physical or sexual abuse < age 18	61.8	73.2	79.2	70.9	NS
Traumatic events in past 6 months	46.3	40.0	43.5	42.3	NS
Generally feel safe[d]					
Moderate or less	20.9	33.3	38.8	30.0	NS
Very safe	58.2	50.9	46.9	51.7	
Extremely safe	20.9	15.8	14.3	18.3	
Main problem substance, self-report					
Alcohol only	10.3	15.8	10.2	11.6	NS
Alcohol with other drug	10.3	7.0	10.2	8.8	NS
Heroin	29.4	43.9	46.9	39.2	NS
Cocaine/crack	38.2	22.8	14.3	27.6	.0113
Other[f]	11.8	10.5	18.4	12.7	NS

Characteristics	Black/African American		Latina		White		Total[e]		P value
	M	SD	M	SD	M	SD	M	SD	
Age in years	36.8	6.7	33.3	6.9	35.3	8.6	35.3	7.5	.0353
Total monthly income	$519	$465	$718	$1,385	$761	$796	$647	$930	NS
Age first alcohol use	15.5	3.9	15.2	3.9	13.7	2.6	14.8	3.6	NS
Age first cocaine/crack use	22.0	5.5	19.8	5.7	18.7	4.4	20.4	5.4	.006
Age first heroin use	21.8	5.9	21.7	7.2	24.7	6.3	22.7	6.5	NS
ASI–alcohol	.12	.25	.12	.23	.07	.18	.10	.22	NS
ASI–drug	.09	.09	.16	.20	.08	.10	.11	.14	.0023
Global Severity Index	1.25	.85	1.78	.81	1.57	.75	1.49	.84	.0017
PSS–Total Score	23.3	13.9	28.5	10.9	26.9	10.9	25.7	12.3	NS

[a] Mutually exclusive Race/Ethnicity groups coded as Hispanic first; if not Hispanic then Black, white or other non-Hispanic
[b] Of those ever had children
[c] Symptoms met criteria for probable psychiatric problem on the Brief Symptom Inventory
[d] In general, how safe do you feel where you currently live?
[e] Includes 7 women who reported other racial/ethnic group or more than 1 race/ethnic group. All totals based on valid N, however, and may be less than 181.
[f] Includes marijuana, other opiates/analgesics, sedatives/benzodiazepines/tranquilizers/hypnotics, other illegal drugs, polydrug, and one respondent reporting no problem.

NOTE: BSI is Brief Symptom Inventory; M is Mean; PSS is Post-traumatic Stress Diagnostic Scale; ASI is Addiction Severity Index.

extremely safe in their current living arrangements than Latina or white women. In the major drug of choice, overall 11.6% identified alcohol use as the major problem and 8.8% reported alcohol in combination with another drug. There was only one group difference: Cocaine/crack was the drug of choice more frequently among African American women while heroin was reported more often among Latina and non-Hispanic White women. Regarding mean age at first use, African American women were more likely to begin use of cocaine/crack at a later age than other groups began their drug use. Drug scores on the Addiction Severity Index (McLellan et al., 1980) were statistically different across groups with Latinas having a higher mean score.

DEVELOPMENT OF THE INTERVENTION

The major goal of the Consortium was to develop and implement an integrated trauma-specific model of alcohol and drug addiction treatment for urban, poor and culturally diverse women with co-occurring mental health disorders and a history of physical and/or sexual abuse that could be useful to other city health departments in large metropolitan areas serving similar populations.

Developmental Research Approach and Findings

During the Phase 1 planning process, a needs assessment was conducted to identify service needs and gaps. Data were collected using a variety of methods including focus groups and in-depth interviews with managers, clinicians, front line staff and Consumers/Survivors, Recovering (CSRs)[2] women from varied service sectors including alcohol and drug addiction treatment, mental health treatment, health and social services, and domestic violence programs. Additional information was obtained from community hearings held by the Boston Public Health Commission and notes from deliberations by Consortium members. The major themes that emerged from the needs assessment (McGraw et al., 2002) are summarized below.

In keeping with other reports of lack of integrated services in alcohol and drug addiction treatment (Grella, 1996), service providers, administrators and consumers characterized the existing system of care as difficult to access and marked by inadequate and fragmented services. Some alcohol and drug abuse treatment programs did not allow women to be on psychotropic medications as evidenced by the following comment from a provider: "Finding a dual diagnosis program first of all, for women, is impossible. I've had a client go off her meds to go into a residential program. . . . She would go off her meds, go extremely acute and flip out there and then they wouldn't let her back in."

Providers noted that other restrictions limited mental health services in the context of the AOD treatment program. A program administrator noted, "I can't get reimbursed for the services of a psychiatrist from the mental health center. I get reimbursed at a substance abuse rate which is probably far too little for what I'm providing." These restrictions meant that for a given patient, her medical, mental health, and AOD problems were treated by different agencies.

The fragmented or disparate nature of services meant that communication among providers within and across different treatment sectors was very difficult at best, often non-existent. There were substantial differences among the AOD treatment programs in terms of their philosophies of care, staffing, and specific services offered. AOD treatment providers had little incentive or structure to facilitate communication with counterparts in mental health services. One consumer observed, "Because you start getting broken up and this one knows a little bit about yourself, this one know a lot about you, this one doesn't know, this one is giving you medication. . . . It gets a little crazy, you know." Another said: "The hardest thing for me is finding what I need in one place. . . . You know, a lot falls in the cracks."

In addition to the lack of coordination and communication, existing services lacked the capacity to screen for and treat a history of violence or abuse. Women complained that providers would often overlook their history. "I've seen women that you'd notice right away that they've been beat up, that they're using drugs. They're going to the hospital and nobody there is paying attention." "They never truly addressed me, they patched me up and sent me on my way."

Most women had children and this affected their course of seeking treatment. Women who wanted services often faced stigmatization and feared losing custody of their children. These fears also made it difficult for them to seek wanted care. "What made me stay quiet was that people panic when you talk about drug use or domestic violence." The problems they encountered facing a system of poorly coordinated, fragmented care for stigmatized illnesses were compounded by the general lack of culturally competent services.

Many of the existing services were often not designed to address problems specific to women. Providers noted, "The model for the treatment of women is the male model." "We need a system which is more inclusive, more family centered and less individual centered." This lack of appropriate services for women in general was further compounded for women of color. One woman said: "You know, if there was some place that I could feel at home, you know, with my own people, I would have stayed, but there is no program like that. Only 'Americanos,' and they're rough. I had already been through them programs and I didn't like them." Women experienced difficulties trusting their providers: "If I feel that a person is being judgmental, if that person really isn't compassionate, I am not going to feel enough trust in them to open up."

In sum, the interviews with individual providers, program directors, and consumers' own voices validated the rationale behind more closely linking mental health, trauma, and AOD services and to directly addressing the impact of childhood and persistent trauma on women's lives. Information from the needs assessment and the deliberations of the Consortium were used to develop the final intervention model.

Role of Consumers/Recovering Persons/Survivors

The Consortium involved CSRs in a variety of ways including participation in the Consortium Steering Committee, workgroups, and needs assessments; hiring of a CSR Coordinator and senior CSR expert consultants; implementation of a CSR-led Women's Leadership Training Institute, and formation of a CSR Integration Roundtable to provide a focused avenue for consumer-based leadership and input. These components are described in further detail in the following section.

System Level Interventions

During Phase 1, strategies were developed to address system-level gaps that contributed to disjointed care for women with co-occurring disorders. Konrad's (1996) service integration framework was used to develop strategies characteristic of a level three system of care (e.g., formalized joint planning, joint funding/shared resources, written interagency agreements, regular meeting of key players, cross training of staff).

Shared Philosophy

The Consortium dedicated significant time in the beginning to discuss and agree on philosophy, principles, and a statement to guide its work. The final agreed-upon mission and philosophy statement is given below:

> The mission of the Boston Consortium of Services for Families in Recovery is to implement an integrated system of care for women and families recovering from drug addiction, mental illness, and physical and/or sexual abuse. Based on existing evidence that has demonstrated the strong link between trauma, mental illness and addiction disorders, we believe that treatment for alcohol and drug addiction needs to include mental health services as well as services to help families be safe and heal from violence. Services should be respectful of consumer rights and be informed by CSR participation. (BCSFR, 1999, p. 1)

Formalized Joint Planning and Regular Meeting of Key Players

The Consortium formed a Steering Committee (SC) comprised of major stakeholders from the following service sectors: AOD treatment, mental health services, domestic violence programs, public health, other key collaborating agencies and consumers. During Phase 1, the SC discussed service needs, planned service integration activities and identified needed policy changes. During Phase 2, the SC focused on discussions of overall issues of service integration across collaborating sites as well as the nuts and bolts of implementation of intervention elements and activities.

Interagency Agreements

Written agreements were developed with collaborating AOD, mental health and public health service agencies that articulated their roles and responsibilities in service integration clinical activities, participation in group meetings, and staff training. Each of the AOD treatment intervention sites received funding for a part-time intervention study liaison responsible for recruitment of participants, implementation of intervention activities, and adherence to study protocols. Similarly, an agreement with the Boston Medical Center (BMC) Department of Psychiatry included funding for a full-time staff person to work with the Consortium.

Shared Resources

Because participating agencies did not individually have the resources needed to develop an integrated system of care, the Consortium developed mechanisms for sharing resources across agencies. For example, through the BMC Department of Psychiatry, a Mental Health/Trauma Service Coordinator acted as a system boundary spanner, conducted diagnostic assessments, and worked collaboratively with AOD treatment providers to develop trauma-informed treatment planning and mental health and trauma service coordination. Also, intervention groups for clients were facilitated by staff across programs allowing for sharing of staff resources, greater flexibility in scheduling of groups and enabling staff to work collaboratively on clinical services.

Cross Training of Staff

Various mechanisms for cross training of staff were implemented: (a) three-day training on AOD, mental health and trauma services integration (BCSFR, 2003a) for a broad array of AOD, mental health, domestic violence, public health and medical service providers; (b) a series of two-hour-long training sessions on integrated trauma-informed systems of care for administrators and managers from collaborating agencies; (c) intensive training on manualized trauma treatment groups; (d) a Service Integration Roundtable luncheon that met quarterly for training and discussions on trauma, mental health and service integration; and (e) establishment of an Interdisciplinary Resource Team (IRT). The IRT meetings were attended by staff from collaborating sites and included a brief lecture by an expert trauma consultant, case presentations by AOD treatment counselors, and discussion about approaches to integrated trauma services relevant to case presentations. A resource document was developed based on the brief trauma integration lecture, case presentation and lessons learned (BCSFR, 2003b).

Individual Level Interventions

The components of the enhanced model were informed by a review of the literature, needs assessment findings, resources available from collaborators, input from consumers and available resources. All services and groups were provided in English and Spanish by trained bilingual and racially/ethnically diverse staff. There were four enhanced service components.

Co-Morbidity Screening

A Co-morbidity Screen developed by the Consortium consisted of items drawn from either published, validated, standard screening tools or from a consensus of CSRs and experts in the field for items not available from validated measures (Liebshutz et al., 2002). An accompanying Co-morbidity Resource Card (BCSFR, 2003c) contained local referral sources for clients and staff. The Co-morbidity Screen was administered as part of the clinical intake process at all participating AOD treatment service sites and a database was developed for ongoing documentation of co-occurring disorders in the service system. A validation study of the screen was recently completed (Amaro et al., 2003).

Diagnostic Assessment, Treatment Planning, and Services Coordination Protocol

A protocol for mental health and trauma diagnostic assessment, treatment planning, and service coordination was implemented by the Mental Health Services Coordinator, who served as a "boundary spanner" between AOD and mental health treatment services. This included conducting trauma/mental health assessments, meeting with AOD treatment counselors to develop trauma-informed treatment plans, making referrals, and coordinating other mental health and trauma treatment services as needed.

Trauma Recovery and Empowerment (TREM) Groups

The Consortium implemented the Trauma Recovery and Empowerment (Harris, 1998), which is a structured manualized trauma treatment psychoeducational approach. Groups were facilitated jointly by two clinicians from different intervention sites to enhance interagency collaboration and training. The TREM model was adapted into a 25-session format that integrated three HIV/AIDS prevention sessions from an empirically tested curriculum (El-Bassel, Hadden & Schilling, 1993). TREM employs a skills building approach to assist women in understanding the link between trauma history, addiction, and sexual risk and provides women with the opportunity to develop positive and protective coping skills to avoid future abuse and strategies for reducing trauma symptoms and sexual risk. The HIV-informed TREM curriculum was translated into Spanish, culturally adapted and pilot tested (BCSFR, 2003d).

Skills-Building Groups

Four trauma-informed skills building groups were provided: (a) Women's Leadership Training Institute (BCSFR, 2003e), a peer-run manualized group intervention comprised of three sessions (15 hours) of intensive training on leadership and communication skills, was developed by the Consortium that focused on the silencing effects of trauma and the process of regaining one's voice; (b) Economic Success in Recovery (BCSFR, 2003f), a manualized skills-based eight-session (2 hours per session) group that assists women with a history of economic dependence on abusive partners in gaining skills to take charge of their finances and to increase skills in dealing with management of money, was adapted by the Consortium from an existing program at a collaborating agency; (c) Pathways to Reunification and Recovery (BCSFR, 2003g), a ten-session (1.5 hours per session) manualized skills-building group that focuses on building skills, information and support related to child custody issues, was adapted by the Consortium from an existing program at a collaborating agency; and (d) Family Nurturing Program (Moore et al., 1995), a twelve-session (2 hours each) manualized skills-building group focusing on parenting skills and family communication.

DESCRIPTION OF INTERVENTION SITES

Five licensed AOD treatment programs located in Boston participated as enhanced intervention sites. The intervention sites were chosen based on their participation during Phase 1 of the project, history of serving Latina and African American women, historical relationship with the Boston Public Health Commission, and willingness to participate in the intervention. At project onset, intervention sites had limited experience in providing trauma-informed and trauma-specific services. All programs had close working relationships with many local social and health care agencies and had some staff in recovery.

Residential AOD Treatment

Three women's residential treatment programs served as intervention sites. *Entre Familia*, a residential AOD treatment facility founded in 1996 by the BPHC, that can serve 23 women and their children, provides 12-month residential treatment to Latina women and their children. The program philosophy stresses gender and culturally specific services guided largely by cognitive behavioral treatment approaches. Its staff is primarily bilingual and bicultural with bachelor and masters training. *Griffin House*, a residential AOD treatment facility founded in 1999 by the Harvard Street Community Health Center with the capacity to serve 24 women and their children, provides 12-month residential treatment primarily to African American women. Although the program philosophy is based on the therapeutic community model with a strong Afro-centric perspective, the program serves women from all racial and ethnic groups. Its staff is largely African American. *Women's Circle*, a residential treatment facility founded by the Harvard Street Community Health Center in 1987 with the capacity to serve 14 women, provides 9-month services primarily to African American women (no children) based on an Afro-centric model. Its staff is largely African American.

Outpatient AOD Treatment Programs

The *Mom's Project Outpatient Program*, an outpatient AOD treatment program, founded in 1988 under the BPHC, serves approximately

80 primarily African American and Latina clients per year. The program philosophy stresses gender and culturally specific approaches guided largely by cognitive behavioral treatment and participatory education approaches. Program staff is largely bilingual (Spanish/English) and bicultural (African American and Latina) with bachelor and masters training. *Substance Abuse Treatment and Prevention (SAPT)-Addiction Services*, a methadone and outpatient treatment program, is part of the BPHC Substance Abuse Services Bureau and has been in existence for 30 years. SAPT provides services to approximately 450 women clients per year. Staff is ethnically diverse and includes bachelor and masters trained counselors, nurses, psychologists, acupuncturist, and physicians.

IMPLEMENTATION CHALLENGES AND LESSONS LEARNED

The Consortium intervention involved collaboration among multiple agencies representing diverse disciplinary perspectives, service foci, and treatment philosophies. Collaborating agencies also varied with respect to infrastructure development, fiscal resources and capacity to integrate new services. Although the diversity of stakeholders made the process of consensus and implementation challenging, it is probably reflective of the collaborations that many community-based service settings would need to achieve for the integration of trauma services. Because all agencies served poor, urban and racially/ethnically diverse populations, the lessons learned in the implementation of the Consortium are likely to be of most relevance to AOD treatment programs serving similar populations.

Obtaining Full Support from Institution's Leadership to Head the Effort

The Consortium faced the *challenge* of overcoming initial apprehension among mid-level managers and front line staff. An important *strategy* was the engagement of leadership from collaborating agencies. Their visibility and support for the project was pivotal in communicating the importance of the project to front line staff and mid-level managers. The Consortium's leadership included the project's principal investigator, who serves as the Vice-Chair of the Board of the BPHC; Director of the Division of Women and Families Substance Abuse Services; Executive Director of the BPHC; clinical directors of the participating programs and key staff from collaborating agencies. These individuals were well placed to support the project team in developing collaborations with key programs and agencies and giving the Consortium high visibility and priority within the institution. An important *lesson* is that for a project of this nature and complexity to be successful, it is essential to count on the full and sustained visible support of the institution's leadership from early stages of project.

Developing Mechanisms for Sustained Communication

Developing and maintaining effective communication among a large group of collaborators was a major *challenge* for the Consortium in all phases of the project. Multiple *strategies* implemented to address communication challenges included: discussions early in the project to arrive at a shared philosophy and mission statement; regular meetings of the Steering Committee; presentations and discussions with the front line staff; memorandums of agreement and contractual agreements with collaborators to clarify roles and responsibilities; newsletters, brochures, informational and educational materials that communicate the intervention philosophy, structure and components; ongoing staff training; and manualized intervention protocols. An important *lesson* is that the process of inter-agency collaboration and the introduction of a new service model need to be approached as a team-building task with emphases in creating systems that foster effective communication, development of a group identity and a shared sense of accountability.

Implementing Multiple and Sustained Approaches for Integration of Consumer Voices

The Consortium faced the *challenge* of integrating CSR participation in a system with few formal mechanisms for engagement of sustained CSR participation and leadership and diverse staff perspectives on the appropriate role of consumer input. The Consortium used multiple *strategies* to achieve CSR integration that included hiring and engaging existing CSR staff at all levels of the organizational structure and implementation of the Consumer Integration Roundtable and CSR Leadership Training Institute. The most important *lesson* on CSR integration is that multiple, sustained and complementary approaches that allow for trial and error are most likely to be successful.

Implementing Effective Workgroup Structures

The Consortium relied on workgroups to carry out important tasks. Reliance on volunteer members from collaborating agencies presented *challenges* to attendance and productivity in completing assigned work. The *strategies* to overcome this challenge included developing clearly defined short-term workgroup tasks and assignment of staff and/or paid consultants to chair workgroups and provide guidance and support. A *lesson* in working with workgroups comprised of volunteer collaborators was to limit the amount of work required by non-paid members and to have staff conduct the background work to assist the group in completing assigned tasks.

Accomplishing Systems Change Through Staff Training

The Consortium faced the *challenge* of implementing system change with staff that lacked an understanding of co-occurring disorders, clinical skills for implementing the interventions and limited initial support for changing services. As a *strategy* to address these challenges, during Phase 1, the Consortium developed a cross-training curriculum focused on the connections among alcohol, and drug addiction, mental illness and history of trauma and the existing barriers to services integration. The cross training was provided to over 80 service providers across diverse systems of care. The initial focus on training a broad group of providers proved helpful in obtaining support for the Consortium's goal of implementing an integrated system. During Phase 2, the Consortium's training became targeted on specific clinical group interventions and clinical strategies for integration of trauma into AOD treatment. An important *lesson* is that intensive and ongoing staff training that addresses provider concerns and enhances clinical knowledge, skills and competencies in treatment of co-occurring disorders is essential to staff engagement and building long-term sustainability of trauma-informed services.

Filling Gaps by Hiring Expert Consultants

Another *challenge* recognized early in the project was that while members of the Consortium had diverse skills that were useful to the group, some skills necessary to carry out the project were not available among collaborators. To address this challenge, the Consortium used the *strategy* of hiring expert consultants to assist in various activities such as the development of the CSR Integration Roundtable, manualized group treatment protocols, provider and consumer educational materials on trauma, training on specific trauma and mental health treatment clinical issues, and professional translation of materials. A *lesson* that might be useful to programs undertaking a similar initiative is to assess early on in the process the expertise needed from external experts and to contract with them to augment the skills of group members.

Engagement of Front Line Staff and Managers in Evaluation Activities

The evaluation of the Consortium's intervention required participation of staff at all levels. Yet, engaging and motivating staff to devote time to completing paperwork related to the implementation of the intervention represented a *challenge* due to the multiple and high demands they faced in delivering services. The *strategies* to address this challenge included combined meetings for project and evaluation staff to provide feedback on findings and progress towards meeting project goals and for evaluators to obtain input and ideas from program staff. One important *lesson* is that it is critical to identify ways to increase staff understanding of the need for evaluation activities and the need for their participation in conducting data collection and other related activities. At the same time, it is also important for evaluation staff to benefit from staff input on methods to improve approaches to data collection that involves program staff.

Development of a Good Client Participation Tracking System

Because the Consortium project involved multiple program sites and intervention components, tracking client participation in various components was a *challenge*. The major *strategy* to address this challenge was the development of a computerized participant tracking system from which reports could be generated to identify client exposure to intervention elements including enrollment, attendance and completion of groups. This system enabled us to have an ongoing accurate assessment of client participation in the intervention so that project staff could better manage client enrollment and engagement, which were essential to achieving the project goals. An important *lesson* is that developing a computerized system for tracking client participation in intervention components is key to the success of any intervention.

Participation and Retention of Clients in the Intervention

The Consortium faced several *challenges* related to participation and retention of clients that varied by treatment modality and program and also by intervention component. For example, because of the structured nature of residential treatment and the availability of clients, program elements were more easily implemented in residential programs. Also, program sites varied with respect to staff resources, infrastructure and internal problems, factors that affected staff availability and degree of active participation in the intervention. Finally, the high drop-out rate in the first months of AOD treatment resulted in lower completion rates for group interventions of longer duration such as TREM. The Consortium employed various *strategies* to address these challenges. Counselors in non-residential programs conducted active outreach to clients including making phone calls and discussing the interventions at standard group and individual group sessions. Although this effort was somewhat effective in the outpatient setting, it was not as effective for the methadone program, which was facing multiple personnel and leadership challenges and whose clients were not accustomed to receiving intensive services. Further, in an effort to increase participation among women who dropped out of treatment, clients were allowed to continue participation in intervention activities after leaving treatment. However, few clients who had dropped out of treatment continued in intervention activities due to relapse, moving out of the area, or seeking services at other agencies. Several important *lessons* emerged. First, highly intensive interventions such as the one implemented by the Consortium may be best suited for residential and intensive outpatient settings. Second, programs facing significant staffing and leadership changes and whose norms are not consistent with the provision of intensive services, may not be ready for implementation of models such as the one implemented by the Consortium. Finally, in the early stages of AOD treatment where high treatment discontinuation rates are common, it may be advisable to offer shorter-term trauma recovery groups as an initial approach to engaging women in trauma recovery work.

Conducting Cultural and Linguistic Adaptation of Treatment Approaches and Materials

Because the target population served by the Consortium was primarily African American and Latina women, the use of existing curricula posed a *challenge* because most had not been translated and others were not culturally adapted. The Consortium utilized the following *strategies* to address this challenge: (a) working groups comprised of African American and Latina group facilitators and a curriculum writer were formed to review and revise existing curricula for cultural appropriateness and relevance based on input from focus groups held with CSRs; (b) a professional translator who is a native Puerto Rican Spanish speaker was hired to conduct a formal translation of the curricula, with translations reviewed by bilingual group facilitators; (c) all revised and translated curricula were pilot tested and final revisions made; and (d) final curricula were formatted and printed for distribution. The most critical *lesson* regarding cultural and linguistic adaptation of curricula is that through a structured and systematic approach, program staff with assistance from expert consultants can produce appropriate curricula for African American and Latina women. It is also important to note that if done properly, cultural and linguistic adaptation of materials is a lengthy and staff intensive process that needs to be planned accordingly. Yet, it is a necessary step in the development of trauma-informed services for ethnically and linguistically diverse populations. (Again, a point for conclusion.)

CONCLUSION

The Boston Consortium of Services for Families in Recovery Model for integrating trauma and mental health services in women's alcohol and/or drug addiction treatment programs provides a useful model for other systems of care serving similar urban populations. Although the program initially faced many obstacles to integration of services, the approaches and strategies employed to address challenges were generally successful and resulted in a more integrated system of mental health, trauma, and alcohol and/or other drug abuse treatment services for the predominantly African American, Latina, poor and urban women served by the Consortium.

As demonstrated in the project's description and implementation process, however, service integration requires commitment from the top leadership among collaborating agencies, a process for engaging staff at all levels in the development of a shared philosophy, and ongoing skills-building training efforts as well as manualized curriculum-based approaches and structured protocols for trauma-specific services. Further, interagency agreements are essential for successful collaboration in the process of systems integration and implementation of mechanisms for involvement and leadership of women in the service population, all essential for lasting systems change. Similarly, successful integration of trauma and mental health services for women of color is not possible without a structured and sustained approach for cultural adaptation and translation of intervention services. This requires collaboration among providers, expert consultants, input from consumers and multiple field testing and revision of manualized curricula.

All of these strategies and approaches require a significant initial investment of time and resources as well a commitment to the ongoing support of mechanism for sustaining an integrated system of care that addresses the needs of women with co-occurring mental illness, trauma and alcohol and/or drug abuse disorders. Although some of the strategies described here may be applicable to other service settings, other systems of care will need to tailor an approach with modifications based on local needs, constraints and resources.

NOTES

1. The U.S. Census considers Hispanic an ethnic group whose members can be of any race.
2. CSR is used to refer to women consumers of mental health services, survivors of trauma and recovering from alcoholism or drug addiction.

REFERENCES

Amaro, H., & Hardy-Fanta, C. (1995). Gender relations in addiction and recovery. *Journal of Psychoactive Drugs, 27*(4), 325-337.
Amaro, H., Lincoln, A., Chernoff, M., Lopez, L. M., & Medrano, L. (2003). *Validation of a Brief Screening Instrument for Identifying Women in Substance Abuse Treatment with Co-occurring Mental Health Problems and Trauma History.* Submitted to the AMERSA National Conference, Baltimore, MD, November 6-8, 2003.
Amaro, H., Navarro, A. M., Conron, K. J., & Raj, A. (2001) Cultural influences on women's sexual health. In: R. J. DiClemente & G. M. Wingood (Eds.), *Women's Sexual & Reproductive Health: Social, Psychological and Public Health Perspectives* (pp. 71-92). New York: Plenum Press.
Amaro, H., Nieves, R., Wolde Johannes, S., & Labault Cabeza, N. (1999). Residential substance abuse treatment with Latinas: Critical issues and challenges. *Hispanic Journal of Behavioral Sciences, 21*(3), 266-282.
Amaro, H., & Raj, A. (2000). On the margin: The realities of power and women's HIV risk reduction strategies. *Journal of Sex Roles, 42*(7/8), 723-749.
Amaro, H., Whitaker, R., Coffman, G., & Heeren, T. (1990). Acculturation and marijuana and cocaine use: Findings from the Hispanic HANES. *American Journal of Public Health, 80*, 54-60.

Bassuk, E. L., Perloff, J. N., & Garcia-Coll, C. (1998). The plight of extremely poor Puerto Rican and White single mothers. *Social Psychiatry and Psychiatric Epidemiology, 33*(7), 326-336.

Beck, A., Karberg, J., & Harrison, P. (2002). *Prison and jail inmates at midyear 2001.* Washington, DC: Bureau of Justice Statistics.

Boston Consortium of Services for Families in Recovery. (1999). *Philosophy and Principles.* Boston Public Health Commission, Boston, MA.

Boston Consortium of Services for Families in Recovery. (2002a). *Spanish Adaptation and Translation of TREM Curriculum.* Boston Public Health Commission, Boston, MA.

Boston Consortium of Services for Families in Recovery. (2003b). *Case-Based Trauma Services Integration Resource Book.* Boston Public Health Commission, Boston, MA.

Boston Consortium of Services for Families in Recovery. (2003c). *Services Resource Card.* Boston Public Health Commission, Boston, MA.

Boston Consortium of Services for Families in Recovery. (2002d). *Spanish Adaptation and Translation of TREM Curriculum.* Boston Public Health Commission, Boston, MA.

Boston Consortium of Services for Families in Recovery. (2002e). *Women's Leadership Training Institute Curriculum.* Boston Public Health Commission, Boston, MA.

Boston Consortium of Services for Families in Recovery. (2002f). *Economic Success in Recovery Curriculum.* Boston Public Health Commission, Boston, MA.

Boston Consortium of Services for Families in Recovery. (2003g). *Pathways to Reunification and Recovery Curriculum.* Boston Public Health Commission, Boston, MA.

Boyd, C. J. (1993). The antecedents of women's crack cocaine abuse: Family substance abuse, sexual abuse, depression and illicit drug use. *Journal of Substance Abuse Treatment, 10*, 433-438.

Brown,V., Huba, G. J., & Mechior, L.A. (1995). Level of burden: Women with more than one co-occurring disorder. *Journal of Psychoactive Drugs, 27*(4), 339-346.

Browne, A. (1991). The victim's experience: Pathways to disclosure. *Psychotherapy: Theory, Research, Practice, Training, 28*(1), 150-156.

Browne, A. (1993). Family violence and homelessness: The relevance of trauma histories in the lives of homeless women. *American Journal of Orthopsychiatry, 63*(3), 370-385.

Browne, A., & Bassuk, S. S. (1997). Intimate violence in the lives of homeless and poor housed women: Prevalence and patterns in an ethnically diverse sample. *American Journal of Orthopsychiatry, 6*, 261-278.

Bureau of the Census. (2002). *Race and Hispanic or Latino Origin by Age and Sex for the United States: 2000 (PHC-T-8).* Retrieved May 5, 2002, from U.S. Census Bureau website: http://www.census.gov/population/cen2000/phc-t08/tab08.pdf

Caetano, R., Cunradi, C. B., Clark, C. L., & Schafer, J. (2000). Intimate partner violence and drinking patterns among White, Black, and Hispanic couples in the U.S. *Journal of Substance Abuse, 11*(2), 213-138.

Chalk, R., & King, P. A. (Eds.) (1998). *Violence in Families: Assessing Prevention and Treatment Programs.* Committee on the Assessment of Family Violence Interventions, National Research Council and Institute of Medicine, Washington, DC: The National Academies.

Derogatis, L. R., & Melisaratos, N. (1983). The Brief Symptom Inventory: An introductory report. *Psychological Medicine, 13*(3), 595-605.

Dutton, M. A., Orloff, L. E., & Aguilar Hass, G. (2000). Characteristics of help-seeking behaviors, resources and service needs of battered immigrant Latinas. *Georgetown Journal on Poverty Law & Policy, 2*(2), 245-305.

Eberstein, I., & Frisbie, W. M. (1976). Differences in marital instability among Mexican Americans, Blacks, and Anglos: 1960 and 1970. *Social Problems, 23*, 609-621.

El-Bassel, N., Hadden, B. R., & Schilling, R. F. (1993). *AIDS Prevention (Skills Building and Relapse) Protocol.* New York, NY: Columbia University School of Social Work.

Foa, E. B., Riggs, D. S., Dancu, C. V., & Rothbaum, B. O. (1993). Reliability and validity of a brief instrument for assessing post-traumatic stress disorder. *Journal of Traumatic Stress, 6*, 459-73.

Fullilove, M., Fullilove, R. E., Haynes, K., & Gross, S. (1990). Black women and AIDS Prevention: A view towards understanding the gender rules. *Journal of Sex Research, 27*(1), 47-64.

Fullilove, M. T., Fullilove, R. E., Smith, M., Winkler, K., Michael, C., Panzar, P. G., & Wallace, R. (1993). Violence, trauma and posttraumatic stress disorder among women drug users. *Journal of Traumatic Stress, 6*, 533-543.

Gelles, R. J., & Conte, J. R. (1990). Domestic violence and sexual abuse of children: A review of research in the eighties. *Journal of Marriage and the Family, 52*, 1045-1058.

Gil-Rivas, V., Fiorentine, R., Anglin, M. D., & Taylor, E. (1997). Sexual and physical abuse: Do they compromise drug treatment outcomes? *Journal of Substance Abuse Treatment, 14*(4), 351-358.

Goodman, L. A., Rosenberg, S. D., Mueser, K. T., & Drake, R. E. (1997). Physical and sexual assault history in women with serious mental illness: Prevalence, impact, treatment, and future directions. *Schizophrenia Bulletin, 23*, 685-696.

Grella, C. E. (1996). Background and overview of mental health and substance abuse treatment systems: Meeting the needs of women who are pregnant or parenting. *Journal of Psychoactive Drugs, 28*(4), 319-343.

Harris, M. (1994). Modifications in the service delivery and clinical treatment for women diagnosed with severe mental illness who are also the survivors of sexual abuse trauma. *Journal of Mental Health Administration, 21*(4), 397-406.

Harris, M. (1998). *Trauma Recovery and Empowerment Manual.* New York: Free Press.

Hien, D., & Scheier, J. (1996). Trauma and short-term outcome for women in detoxification. *Journal of Substance Abuse Treatment, 13*, 227-231.

Jasinski. J. L. (1996). *Structural inequalities, family and cultural factors, and spousal violence among Anglo and Hispanic Americans.* Unpublished Doctoral Dissertation, University of New Hampshire, Durham.

Kaufman Kantor, G., Jasinski, J. L., & Aldarondo, E. (1994). Sociocultural status and incidence of marital violence in Hispanic families. *Violence and Victims, 9*(3), 207-222.

Kilpatrick, D. G., Acierno, R., Saunders, B., Resnick, H. S., & Best, C. L. (1997). A 2-year longitudinal analysis of the relationships between violent assault and substance use in women. *Journal of Consulting and Clinical Psychology, 65*(5), 834-847.

Konrad, E. (1996). A multidimensional framework for conceptualizing human services integration initiatives. In Marquart, J., & Konrad, E. (Eds.), *Evaluating Initiatives to Integrate Human Services. New Directions for Evaluation* (pp. 5-19). San Francisco, CA: Jossey-Bass.

Liebshulz, J., Mulvey, K., & Samet, J. (1997). Victimization among substance abusing women. *Archives of General Medicine, 157*, 1093-1097.

Liebshutz, J. M., Lincoln, A., Dooley, J., Amaro, H., & Lopez, L. (2002) *Implementing brief screening for co-occurring mental health symptoms, substance abuse, and trauma history: Tools and strategies.* Poster Presentation at the 130th Annual Meeting of APHA. Philadelphia, PA. November 11th, 2002.

Marin, B. V., Gomez, C. A., Tschann, J. M., & Gregorich, S. E. (1997). Condom use in unmarried Latino men: A test of cultural constructs. *Health Psychology, 16*(5), 458-467.

McCauley, J., Kern, D., Koloder, K., Dill, L., Schroeder, A. F., DeChant, H. K., Ryden, J., Derogatis, L. R., & Bass, E. B. (1997). Clinical characteristics of women with a history of childhood abuse. *Journal of the American Medical Association, 277*, 1362-1368.

McGraw, S. A., Larson, M. J., Ramirez, C., & Belisle, M. (2001). *A qualitative description of the barriers to, and gaps in, treatment for women with co-occurring substance abuse, mental illness and a history of trauma in Boston, MA.* Prepared for the Boston Consortium of Services for Families in Recovery by the New England Research Institutes, Watertown, MA.

McLellan, A. T., Luborsky, L., Woody, G. E., & O'Brien, C. P. (1980). An improved diagnostic evaluation instrument for substance abuse patients: The Addiction Severity Index. *Journal of Nervous Mental Disorders, 168*, 26-33.

Moore, J., Buchan, B., Finkelstein, N., & Thomas, K. (1995). *Nurturing Program for Families in Substance Abuse Treatment and Recovery.* Park City, UT: Family Development Resources, Inc.

Najavits, L. M., Weiss, R. D., & Shaw, S. R. (1997). The link between substance abuse and post traumatic stress disorder in women. *American Journal of Addictions, 6*(4), 273-283.

Okamura, A., Heras, P., & Wong-Kerberg, L. (1995). Asian, Pacific Island, and Filipino Americans and sexual child abuse. In L. A. Fontes (Ed.), *Sexual Abuse in Nine North American Cultures: Treatment and Prevention* (pp. 67-96). Thousand Oaks, CA: Sage Publications.

Perilla, J. A., Bakeman, R., & Norris, F. H. (1994). Culture and domestic violence: The ecology of abused Latinas. *Violence and Victims, 9*(4), 325-339.

Poulsny, M. A., & Follete, V. M. (1995). Long-term correlates of child sexual abuse: Theory and review of the empirical literature. *Applied Preventive Psychology, 4*, 143-166.

Reiger, D. A., Farmer, M. E., Rae, D. S., Locke, B. Z., Keith, S. J., Judd, L. L., & Goodwin, F. K. (1990). Comorbidity of mental disorders with alcohol and other drug abuse. *Journal of the American Medical Association, 264*, 2511-2518.

Romero, G. J., Wyatt, G. E., Loeb, T. B., Carmona, J. V., & Solis, B. M. (1999). The prevalence and circumstances of child sexual abuse among Latina women. *Hispanic Journal of Behavioral Sciences, 21*(3), 351-365.

Senturia, K., Sullivan, M., Ciske, S., & Shiu-Thornton, S. (2000). *Cultural issues affecting domestic violence service utilization in ethnic and hard to reach populations.* Washington, DC: National Institute of Justice/NCJRS.

Sorenson, S. B. (1996). Violence against women: Examining ethnic differences and commonalities. *Evaluation Review, 20,* 123-145.

Sorenson, S. B., & Telles, C. A. (1991). Self-reports of spousal violence in a Mexican-American and non-Hispanic white population. *Violence and Victims, 6,* 3-15.

Substance Abuse and Mental Health Services Administration (SAMHSA). (2002). *Substance Abuse Treatment: Addressing the Special Needs of Women. Treatment Improvement Protocol.* (in preparation).

Sullivan, J. M., & Evans, K. (1994). Integrated treatment for the survivor of childhood trauma who is chemically dependent. *Journal of Psychoactive Drugs, 26*(4), 369-437.

The Sentencing Project. (2003). *Hispanic Prisoners in the United States.* Retrieved May 5, 2002, from The Sentencing Project Website: http://www.sentencingproject.org/brief/pub1051.pdf

Tjaden, P., & Thoennes, N. (2000). *Full report of the prevalence, incidence, and consequences of violence against women.* Report from the National Institute of Justice and the Centers for Disease Control and Prevention, Washington, DC: U.S. Department of Justice.

United States Centers for Disease Control and Prevention. (2001). *HIV/AIDS Surveillance Report, 13(2).* Retrieved May 5, 2002 from CDC Website: http://www.cdc.gov/hiv/stats/hasr1302.pdf

West, C. M. (1998). Lifting the "political gag order": Breaking the silence around partner violence in ethnic minority families. In J. L. Jasinski & L. M. Williams (Eds.), *Partner Violence: A Comprehensive Review of 20 Years of Research* (pp. 184-209). Thousand Oaks, CA: Sage Publications.

West, C. M., Kaufman Kantor, G., & Jasinski, J. L. (1998). Sociodemographic predictors and cultural barriers to help-seeking behavior by Latina and Anglo American battered women. *Violence and Victims, 13*(4), 361-375.

Wingood, G. M., & DiClemente, R. J. (2000). Application of the theory of gender and power to examine HIV-related exposures, risk factors, and effective interventions for women. *Health Education & Behavior, 27*(5), 539-56.

The Portal Project:
A Layered Approach to Integrating Trauma into Alcohol and Other Drug Treatment for Women

Sharon Cadiz, EdD
Andrea Savage, PhD
Diane Bonavota, MSW
James Hollywood, MSW
Erica Butters, MSW
Michelle Neary, MSW
Laura Quiros, MSW

SUMMARY. Palladia, Inc. is a not-for-profit, multi-service agency, located in New York City, serving primarily African-American and Latino communities. Palladia's Portal Project, in collaboration with the evaluation team from Hunter College School of Social Work (HCSSW), participated in the national Women, Co-Occurring Disorders and Violence study. We studied 270 women with co-occurring issues of alcohol and other drug (AOD) problems and mental illness, who had histories of violence, and were high end users of service. Palladia built an integrated

Sharon Cadiz is affiliated with Project Return Foundation, Inc. Andrea Savage is affiliated with Hunter College. Diane Bonavota, James Hollywood, Erica Butters, Michelle Neary, and Laura Quiros are all affiliated with the Portal Project.

[Haworth co-indexing entry note]: "The Portal Project: A Layered Approach to Integrating Trauma into Alcohol and Other Drug Treatment for Women." Cadiz, Sharon et al. Co-published simultaneously in *Alcoholism Treatment Quarterly* (The Haworth Press, Inc.) Vol. 22, No. 3/4, 2004, pp. 121-139; and: *Responding to Physical and Sexual Abuse in Women with Alcohol and Other Drug and Mental Disorders: Program Building* (ed: Bonita M. Veysey, and Colleen Clark) The Haworth Press, Inc., 2004, pp. 121-139. Single or multiple copies of this article are available for a fee from The Haworth Document Delivery Service [1-800-HAWORTH, 9:00 a.m. - 5:00 p.m. (EST). E-mail address: docdelivery@haworthpress.com].

http://www.haworthpress.com/web/ATQ
Digital Object Identifier: 10.1300/J020v22n03_07

system of care and implemented a comprehensive trauma-informed intervention that is designed to put trauma and safety first to assist women in remaining in treatment. Primacy of trauma in the early stages of treatment constitutes a major philosophical shift within the traditional residential drug treatment setting. The focus of the engagement and treatment process is on the role of trauma in the woman's life and its relationship to patterns of AOD abuse and mental illness. Another key feature of the Portal model is the emphasis on normalizing the adaptations which the women have made in response to interpersonal traumatic life events. The women feel less stigmatized and isolated. They are encouraged to see their former coping and adaptive behaviors as strengths rather than maladaptive weaknesses, deficiencies or character flaws. Support for the women in their parenting and family roles and attention to their individual perceptions of culture are also part of the intervention. Portal blends service intervention, policy development, research, and evaluation for effective service delivery. The collaborative work of this project has produced a replicable model that configures specific direct service enhancements and service system improvements, using the active involvement of consumers, practitioners, service providers and policy makers. *[Article copies available for a fee from The Haworth Document Delivery Service: 1-800-HAWORTH. E-mail address: <docdelivery@haworthpress.com> Website: <http://www.HaworthPress.com> © 2004 by The Haworth Press, Inc. All rights reserved.]*

KEYWORDS. Alcoholism, drug abuse, women, physical abuse, sexual abuse, integration, urban

INTRODUCTION

Palladia, Inc. is an organization with over thirty years of experience in the field of alcohol and drug treatment. Palladia has designed and implemented the Portal Project, an innovative approach that intervenes with the complex issues of trauma, AOD problems and mental illness as they occur among a female, addicted population within a residential drug treatment setting. The program developed an infrastructure and organizational resources to treat and study the targeted women. This unique design for care and investigation evolved, over a five-year period, into an influential model for addressing one of the most challenging issues confronting addicted women and related systems of care; namely, trauma and its various manifestations.

Alcohol and drug treatment alone cannot always explain or detect the complex interplay and causality linking patterns of addiction to antecedent life experiences of childhood abuse, loss, abandonment, maltreatment, and episodic or long-term interpersonal violence. Using a trauma framework, it is possible to more clearly identify the role and roots of addiction, as well as strengthen recovery interventions for women.

A substantial body of literature establishes the fact that women are uniquely burdened and beset by multiple issues and vulnerabilities that impede their process of treatment and recovery. These challenges are often barriers for women seeking help and can contribute to early departure from treatment and relapse. The Portal Project consists of a mobile clinical team, program services staff, and a research team. The mission is to respectively effect change on the levels of direct service, practice and policy related to the problem and investigate the outcomes and impact of these applied methods and approaches. The women were from inner city communities in and around New York City. They entered treatment at two of Palladia's residential drug treatment programs.

The history of Palladia provides additional evidence that early efforts to address the needs of women within traditional drug treatment settings creates organizational as well as individual challenges that are not easily resolved. Not long after Palladia's primarily male therapeutic community was established, women suffering from addiction began entering treatment. However, it was soon discovered that women were often intimidated by a male-dominated treatment setting. They also had exclusive needs and concerns different from their male counterparts. Therefore, a female-focused treatment strategy was developed and over time integrated into the existing program to meet their needs. Palladia took a series of steps to lift the stigma for women struggling with addiction to normalize the treatment needs of women, and to lay a foundation in gender-specific work that was further developed by the Portal Project.

A preliminary finding from case readings done in the beginning phase of the project revealed that in a majority of the cases trauma was not treated prior to entering treatment, and was not significantly addressed in treatment plans.

The Portal Project's layered approach to integrating trauma into the treatment environment consists of enhanced assessment, direct services, multidisciplinary team case conferences, consumer participation, and collaborative cross-system policy and planning work.

The layered approach refers specifically to the layers of intervention that are organized to have an impact on multiple problems. The women's lives represent complex networks of contacts, relationships, and problems that are interconnected. Layering enhances the quality of care for individuals who must seek help in multiple service systems. By creating layers of staff, multidisciplinary practitioners, and policy makers the project is able to fold in diverse service enhancements, problem solve issues on different levels and keep the process open to multiple collaborators while maintaining a responsiveness to environmental changes.

STATEMENT OF THE PROBLEM

Women develop in connection to others, embedded in a web of relationships. Healthy childhood development permits women to gain self-esteem, empowerment, and connections. Experiences of trauma, especially childhood physical and sexual abuse, affect the development process and connections causing an interruption in family ties, poor body image, decreased sense of safety and support, and low self-esteem; factors which can stay with women throughout their lives.

Women with AOD problems and mental health disorders and histories of violence have a complex set of issues with which to cope. The lifestyle of alcohol and drug use and related homelessness can exacerbate the trauma, and pose serious threats to safety with increased chances of reassault, both sexual and physical. There exists the danger of exchanging sex or money for drugs and the threat of HIV/AIDS due to unprotected sex. Incarceration remains a reality for many of these women; 60% of our women have been incarcerated and mandated to treatment. Many have been in environments difficult for trauma survivors, especially in terms of hypervigilance and dangers of re-traumatization; and many have been separated from their children.

A central issue for our women is their risk of loss of connection to their children and the challenge of reconnection. AOD abuse often leads to incarceration, reports to child welfare about the safety of the children, and removal of the children. This is all compounded by the reality that these women have fractured support networks and are often forced to be in contact with those who abused them or who did not protect them. Often, these same people are involved with their children.

Trauma is ubiquitous in the lives of women with AOD and mental health disorders, and remains the "elephant in the room" in the drug treatment world. The ongoing question in residential treatment programs is when to address the trauma and its issues. Residential drug treatment programs often do not deal with trauma issues early on in treatment for fear that women will relapse. Without diagnosis and treatment of trauma, female alcohol and drug abusers are vulnerable to relapse and or revictimization (Bollerud, 1990). Feedback from consumers in focus groups shows women feel silenced again and required to "keep the secret" about trauma when discouraged from talking about it too early in their treatment.

The need for integrated services for women has been well documented by the literature, consumer input, reports conducted by federal agencies, program staff experience, and findings from internal and external studies. In the initial phase of the Portal Project study, focus groups conducted at program sites with consumers and Multi-Disciplinary Team Case Conferences document the complexity of women's needs and the failure of a single set of program-specific services. Consumers identified the following issues: long waiting periods for available space, being treated like a victim, lack of specialty groups, child placement in foster care, and the need for a higher regard for services that include consumer involvement and peer support.

When women enter the residential treatment "portal," there is a low probability that in the 6- to 12-month stay, all of their issues and needs will be addressed and met. Women with co-occurring AOD and mental health disorders with histories of trauma and their dependent children must deal with systems and service providers that typically compartmentalize the care and attention provided to address their multiple needs. Konrad (1996) refers to categorical barriers, inherent difficulties within nonintegrated systems and barriers to integration efforts as principle challenges facing many service systems. 12-Step programs can be retraumatizing and shaming for both male and female survivors of trauma. Perceived coercion or forced choices within the treatment setting can cause clients to re-experience an earlier trauma or undergo a new traumatic experience. From a mental health perspective, client behaviors in response to power imbalances can be labeled pathological when they actually represent adaptations and coping methods in response to earlier trauma.

The Portal Project documented the critical components of an integrated system: peer and consumer involvement, gender-specific services, culturally competent practices, cross-training attention to trauma, multidisciplinary team approach, and a dual focus on co-occurring disorders. Gender specific treatment includes a strength based, non-confrontational, safe, nurturing and supportive environment. Multidisciplinary team models, bringing together professionals from different fields to develop a holistic portrait of the client, are essential for an integrated system of care.

The Portal model recognizes that the issue of gender exists within many contexts: race, culture, age, sexual orientation, socioeconomic, class, ability, living situation, health status, and motherhood. In working with people with ADM disorders and related syndromes, integrating treatment approaches to improve the chances for a successful outcome is critical (Kofed, Friedman & Peck, 1993; Sullivan & Evans, 1994). An integrated treatment approach means conceptualizing the two syndromes of AOD problems and mental illness as independent co-existing disorders, assessing clients for the presence of the disorders simultaneously (Sullivan & Evans, 1994), and understanding the diversity of substance-using and abusing women.

Because women are embedded in a web of complex relationships, made even more complex by early abuse and trauma, it is crucial to attend to these relationships during treatment. Treatment should assist clients in understanding these relations, developing skills to cope with those that are most problematic and developing skills to expand their friends and supportive ties. The residential alcohol and drug treatment setting provides a safe environment in contrast to the living conditions the clients may have had before, limits the threat of physical and sexual abuse, a break from alcohol and drug use and the lifestyle, offers a respite from child care which may permit the women to focus on her needs, and limits contact with those in her family and support network who may have been involved in her trauma. The women report challenges they face when they revisit the trauma once drug-free. Although implicitly a safe environment, the congregate care setting of the residential drug treatment center presents many challenges for the woman with a history of trauma. Perceived danger and concerns about children and other relationships can sometimes increase the risk of relapse, heighten feelings of isolation, threaten reunification, erode self-esteem and trigger episodes of post-traumatic stress disorder.

TARGET POPULATION

The women in Palladia are female clients from the five boroughs of New York City, and approximately 98% of the women are welfare eligible, 60% have criminal justice issues, 60% have health problems, approximately 11% have HIV/AIDS, 80% have children, about 50% have a high school diploma, and 40-50% are homeless when they first receive services. Palladia serves an estimated 1,000 people a day throughout its programs.

The integrated care settings that comprise the Portal Project are two of Palladia's programs: Starhill Residential Drug Treatment Program and Dreitzer Women and Children's Residential Treatment Center. The usual care setting was Palladia's Willow Avenue Homeless Shelter. The women in the integrated care setting had an average age of 34; 62% were African American, 8% white, 29.4% other; 41% were of Hispanic origin, 24.6% were Puerto Ricans and small numbers (1-4) of Cubans, Mexicans and other Hispanics. One hundred percent of the women had an addiction history, with 71% using crack or cocaine as the primary drug and alcohol as the second most used drug. Sixty-five percent were daily users. Seventy-three percent had a trauma history with 30% childhood sexual or physical abuse; 25% were victims of domestic violence. In terms of mental health history, 27% attempted suicide and 85% reported mental health difficulties. Eighty-five percent had at least one child, with an average of 3 children. Thirty-six percent of clients' children were involved in the child welfare system prior to treatment entry, 64.2% were with family/unrelated others. Twenty-two percent of the women were homeless and living in homeless shelters before entering treatment. The rest came from other treatment services or institutions.

PURPOSE AND GOALS

The purpose and goals focused on testing the Portal model of integrated, gender-sensitive, culturally competent service that pays concurrent attention to the multiple domains of trauma, AOD problems, mental health and parenting; maintaining effective service integration that informs practice and policy while empowering and integrating consumers.

Individual and system level change were major goals of the Portal Project. The underlying purpose for selecting the intervention design and integration strategy stemmed from the understanding that the women would have greater treatment success if the system of care underwent concurrent service changes to address gaps, barriers and service delivery methods.

DEVELOPMENT OF THE INTERVENTION

Developmental Research

A variety of site specific studies were planned to supplement the cross-site study including process evaluation; a multi-method approach including observations of meetings, stakeholder interviews, analysis of documents, work plan analysis, and extensive record reviews to assure that all elements of the model criteria were met at both integrated care and usual care sites. Additionally, client interviews, multi-site narrative interviews, case record reviews and fidelity studies based on observations of treatment groups were developed for the Portal Project evaluation.

The initial phase of the development of the Portal Project outlined the variety and interconnectedness of gender-specific needs in alcohol and other drug treatment programs. In profiling a sample of the women who come through Palladia's programs, the need for an integrated system of care became apparent. The primary issues affecting women entering Palladia's AOD treatment programs were past and present traumatic experiences, mental illness and childcare or parenting concerns. It became clear that not only would several different treatment philosophies needs to be applied in order to treat the whole client and address all of her service needs, but several layers of services, going beyond direct practice would need to be established as well. Implementation of clinical interventions were crucial, but policy, administrative, and peer run domains also needed to be targeted for a truly comprehensive and individualized plan that bridged the gaps in service women in recovery so often face.

Early on in the development of the intervention, emphasis was placed on the integration of the intervention into already existing treatment. The treatment setting had a strong behaviorally based milieu approach that has a long-standing history of difficulty adapting to new perspectives of human development. The integration was achieved by having the Women's Treatment Specialist become part of the treatment team on the unit. She attended staff meetings where case planning was discussed. By attending these meetings she was able to understand the treatment team's perspective of the treatment needs for the client as well as gain an understanding of the overall treatment environment. Placing the Women's Treatment Specialist on the team enabled her to inform the staff of the impact of trauma on human development. This helped the staff develop a broader perspective of the client's needs and underscored the value of having the Trauma Services integrated into the existing treatment.

In addition to being on the Treatment Team, the Women's Treatment Specialist also co-led the group interventions with the mental health staff already employed at the intervention site. This achieved three things: taught the existing staff about the intervention so that they could carry on the groups, enabled more flexibility in leadership (i.e., group could continue even if there was a staff absence), and lastly co-leadership helped the clients to have more options for seeking staff support after group when trauma issues may arise.

System Level

The intervention functioned on various system levels. The intervention site represented a system, along with the community of service providers, and related service systems. System level integration for the Portal Project consisted of two key interventions: (a) monthly Multi-Disciplinary Team Case Conferences (MDTCC) and (b) quarterly Policy Action Committee (PAC) meetings. Each served to address the system level needs of the target population. The purpose of the MDTCC was to assemble expertise and representation from multiple service arenas; facilitate access to services from a variety of agencies and systems; foster positive change in the service delivery and practice areas; maximize information sharing and identify gaps and barriers to service. The PAC was designed to identify structural barriers and gaps in services among multiple systems. A core group of collaborators attended quarterly meetings with the aim of enacting policy changes that were supportive of the integrated treatment approach. Each participating agency or system could designate one or two representatives to attend the monthly MDTCC, in addition to having a policy level administrator at the quarterly PAC meetings. The focus of the committee was to review regulatory policy and funding framework for the service systems which treat women with co-occurring disorders of chemical dependency and mental illness and histories of violence or trauma.

PHILOSOPHIES AND PRINCIPLES

A prominent philosophy of this project and intervention is to treat a person from a holistic perspective; she is not a diagnosis, a trauma victim, or an alcoholic or addict, but a person, a mother, a friend, a daughter. Her diagnoses are only part of who she is or how she behaves. She has many needs that stem from the presenting problem that led her to treatment. Although the women may have similar diagnoses and are addicted to the same substances, each has her own set of unique needs. Treatment needs to be individualized and clinicians needs to be flexible with their approaches. Furthermore, strengths-based language, along with a skills development focus are recommended to help generate an appreciation for resiliency while nurturing an improvement in coping skills. The women are referred to as survivors, not victims, and they are guided in the development of safe coping techniques.

Understanding of trauma-specific dynamics and how they impact those with AOD abuse histories needed to be integrated into the treatment program. This does not translate into merely hiring a trauma specialist, but training of all of the existing staff to help them to become aware of behaviors and symptoms of severe trauma and taking these ideas into account when developing individualized treatment plans. The Portal Project helped to convey the collective understanding that there is no single recipe or formula for recovery. Treatment plans should not look like replicas of one another but should be designed to reflect the unique needs of the individual.

Networking among AOD counselors, mental health providers and trauma specialists is a key element to providing competent integrated care. Communication among professionals is essential to gain further insight into what a client needs and to have the ability to consider another's recommendations when preparing a treatment plan. Conflicting or puritanical treatment philosophies can serve to confuse and frustrate clients, thereby increasing the possibility of relapse.

Lifestyles that often surround addiction, especially for minority women tend to include homelessness, incarceration, violence and prostitution. Many women admitted using alcohol and other drugs as a way to cope with interpersonal traumas in childhood or adulthood. Some women also used substances to cope with mental illnesses such as depression or psychotic disorders. Therefore, relapse carries with it a connotation of revictimization because for these women the two are so often interconnected.

DESCRIPTION OF THE INTERVENTIONS

The intervention took place in two 6- to 12-month long-term residential alcohol and other drug treatment programs: Starhill, a 417-bed co-ed facility, and Dreitzer, a 25-bed facility for mothers with one child. Both were drug-free settings. The program design was milieu therapy employing the Therapeutic Community (TC) approach with a mix of paraprofessional and professional staff administering various interventions. The intervention was developed as an adjunct to the existing treatment that consisted of milieu therapy, individual counseling and psycho-educational groups addressing AOD issues, educational and vocational counseling. The intervention begins in the admissions phase of treatment when the client is identified by the admissions staff as being a candidate for the project and referred for a screening. The client is screened while she is in the orientation phase of treatment. Intervention occurs in the main treatment phase.

Many of the women in treatment are separated from their children. Even the women in the Dreitzer program who had a child with them in treatment also had other children they were separated from by way of foster care or adoption due to termination of parental rights. This separation often surfaces as traumatic loss for these women that they need to process with other women in the program and with their clinicians as well. Consumer support was also helpful to inspire hope and empowerment among clients who feel little hope of reunification with their children or of a successful treatment outcome. Policy meetings bring the philosophy of an integrated treatment approach to other service providers in the community as well as within Palladia's other sites that are not part of the Portal Project. Finally, the introduction of a trauma perspective into treatment facilities for chemical addiction begins to shape the perceptions of clinical and AOD counselors alike, as well as shape administration's treatment approaches for dually diagnosed clients who have profound trauma histories.

The *Cultural Competence Performance Measures for Behavioral Healthcare Programs* (1998) was used as a foundation for the development of the Portal Project's approach to culture. It cites some fundamental cultural issues such as the fact that there are diversities across and within cultural groups. Also, it highlights both misdiagnosis and higher rates of mental health diagnosis among African American and Latina clients partially due to a lack of sensitivity to cultural differences among clinicians. Social stigma associated with mental illness and AOD problems are part of a cultural context and can become a deterrent to those seeking help. Stigma may increase feelings of shame. Systems of care can be viewed as hostile if they don't understand and appreciate traditional ways that cultural groups regard the problem. Other important factors are the need for proximity of the program to the population served and coordinated services delivered by staff attuned to the culture.

The Portal Project addressed culture through an individualized regard for each woman's cultural experience. Assessment and observation of the women in groups and individual sessions served to provide the Portal staff with information about the their beliefs and values. For example, distrust of other women was a commonly expressed belief. It was as much a cultural belief as a social and economic reality experienced by a significant number of the women. They spoke about competition and betrayal that caused them to distrust other women. Case conferencing uncovered key preferences and meanings associated with what helped and hurt, as well as who they trusted and sought out for help. One case presented a Latina woman who only worked with a Latina clinician. The woman refused help from other members of the staff. Consequently, the clinician was repeatedly called at all hours to assist with problems that arose with the woman in the residential treatment setting. Gradually the woman was able to build trust and accept help from other members of staff and utilize the group to process issues. It was concluded that the identification she had with the clinician was driven by a cultural connection based on language, gender and similar background. The culturally sensitive staff knew not to force the woman to make a rapid adjustment. Instead the clinician brought the matter to a case conference and asked for supportive ways to wean the woman away from this exclusive relationship in order to cultivate feelings of trust with other staff and peers. The staff knew that this primary relationship helped the woman to feel safe and it would have had a detrimental effect on the quality of her care if she were forced to make an abrupt change. This is indicative of the type of individualizing that is done using the cultural context for guidance.

Efforts were made to address culture by integrating the service within the familiar setting of the residential treatment facility. By bringing the service to the women and engaging them in a familiar, safe environment, the women were more receptive to the services and the staff. The Women's Treatment Specialists initiated pre-group contact in individual sessions, special orientation groups and introductory meetings. Also, gender-specific, trauma-centered groups minimized stigma through normalizing their experience, giving them identification with others with similar histories, using strengths-based language and supporting and nurturing them with encouragement and simple gestures such as refreshments for meetings. The cultural value of food should not be underestimated. The staff was careful not to present the food and refreshments as a hand out, but as a respectful offering of hospitality. Together these approaches enhanced the quality of the care, made inter-cultural communication more effective, and assisted the engagement process.

It is difficult to understand the complex dynamics of addiction, mental illness and trauma without addressing trauma histories in treatment. However, as safety is the underlying principle in this intervention, the clinical assessments and group interventions with clients have to be very delicate. A trauma group alone if not done skillfully could re-traumatize clients. Therefore, trauma processing was generally done in individual sessions with Women's Treatment Specialists rather than in the group, while the group focused on internalizing a sense of safety and coping skills. The safety of all group members is important. Women can be "triggered" by experiences in group as well as in the larger community. Trauma-informed clinicians are therefore necessary to be able to identify traumatic responses and behavior and make sure members are safe before they leave.

Many of the basic philosophies of a traditional therapeutic community conflict with philosophies about how to treat trauma and what a survivor needs to recover. Re-traumatization, a unilateral treatment approach and minimal use of a strength-based perspective are some of the barriers for women in getting all of their treatment needs met in a residential therapeutic community setting. Encounter groups and the typical philosophies of confrontation and accepting responsibility can be shaming and re-traumatizing for many survivors. Encouraging a trauma survivor with a mental health diagnosis to disclose abuse history in a large co-ed group setting could be detrimental. It can cause more fragile clients to decompensate, either resulting in severe depression or suicidal tendencies, psychosis or severe PTSD symptoms such as dissociation, hypervigilance or flashbacks. Without appropriate crisis intervention these clients are extremely vulnerable to relapse, which for many leads them back to a potentially traumatizing lifestyle. Accountability strategies, such as enforcing a "closed house" can also be re-traumatizing for clients, especially for survivors of domestic violence or child abuse who have memories of being trapped or restrained. The lack of privacy in many residential communities also can be confusing or intrusive to a trauma survivor who has difficulty establishing appropriate boundaries.

Clients making the difficult adjustment to residential treatment, and processing all of the mistakes that they made, need to be able to also focus on what they do that is right and what their strengths are. Working from a strength-based perspective is one treatment approach that may be underused but is essential in working with trauma survivors. Empowerment is an important aspect of trauma work and is something not always found in AOD treatment facilities.

Residential facilities can provide substantial advantages to an integrated treatment approach. Many now provide a multidisciplinary staff which includes psychiatrists and social workers in addition to drug and alcohol counselors. It should also include a multicultural and culturally competent staff that can take cultural implications of mental illness, drug and alcohol dependency and trauma into account. It can be regarded as a safe place, and is often safer than many of the environments clients have been living in prior to coming to treatment. Additionally, trauma-informed staff can make the environment safer for all clients by providing crisis intervention, safety and coping skills for residents. Dreitzer Center, with its all-female population and close-knit setting which provides a smaller counselor to client ratio, may serve to provide a safer experience for some clients. Within the residential setting as well as within individual therapy and groups, clients are supposed to learn to relate safely to one another and the staff, work through feelings rather than acting on them and develop coping skills which serves to create a safer environment for everyone.

From the time a woman first comes in contact with the Portal Project intervention until the time she completes treatment, her service needs are tracked and assessed. The clinical trauma assessment at the beginning helps her to communicate her experience in a safe way as well as validating her and bearing witness to her experience. The clinical group intervention of Seeking Safety, a cognitive behavioral present focused therapy that helps to attain safety from both PTSD and AOD abuse, further addresses her trauma while simultaneously addressing her chemical dependence, their connection and alternative ways to cope. Peer-run services allow her to relate to other women in a supportive way and gain encouragement from peers who have had similar experiences. Other peer-led groups and a peer council continue with consumer coordination to foster the women's connection to recovery and one another. PAC meetings and MDTCC meetings foster change and awareness on the policy and outreach front, and consumers are invited to attend and offer input into enhancing service delivery. Portal Project Women's Treatment Specialists initiated the implementation of a trauma-focused intervention into Starhill and Dreitzer Center using trauma assessment and Seeking Safety group intervention.

ROLE OF CONSUMERS/RECOVERING PERSONS/SURVIVORS

Palladia's growth and success as an agency stems from a long-standing commitment to the role of consumers/recovering persons in reviewing, developing, and shaping standards of care, and identifying gaps in services and reconfiguration. The design of Portal Project focuses on the integration of consumers. Consumer involvement in the project emphasizes values of empowerment, choice and self-determination. Consumers are directly involved in program and policy planning. Consumers who have lived with addiction and trauma have special expertise and insight into the complexity of the needs of women in recovery.

Consumer integration and involvement are present on all levels: from the individual, to the program, organizational and cross-system. The individual level relates to having trauma specific issues integrated into the women's treatment plans. This level of integration promotes a sense of consumer empowerment. On the organizational/program level consumers participate in case conferences, facilitate groups, give input into policy and planning through special meetings and focus groups. Leadership, advocacy training, group facilitation skills and consumer organizing are among the types of assistance offered to the clients involved in the project. Peer-run group facilitation provides role models for consumers within a forum designed for peer interaction. Several peer-run group interventions are utilized in the Portal model. Additionally, the outreach counselor works among consumers in the integrated condition to mobilize and promote involvement, voice and representation in all aspects of service integration and delivery. Peer-run group facilitation provides role models for consumers within a forum designed for peer interaction. The Peer Council provides the participants with the opportunity to build leadership skills and work-related skills. Consumers utilize the group to create and share their voice as women in recovery. The Peer Council is facilitated by the peer outreach counselor and monthly meetings are held addressing mutual support, information needs and activity planning. The Peer Council strengthens efforts to sustain the active role of consumers. The Consumer Advisory Committee (CAC) was created to receive input from the consumers on design and refinement of the evaluation design. In addition, the CAC created a safe space for consumers to share their stories early in treatment as well as at termination and after treatment. The evaluation and narrative gave voice to consumers' views and situations and their treatment experience, providing valuable information to better understand how they got to where they are. A consumer led group for clients followed the Seeking Safety clinical group intervention. It assisted women in developing an understanding of basic safety, while promoting skills that enhance their ability to maintain safety and sobriety, and focuses on interpersonal skills and self-care.

LESSONS LEARNED

Clinical Observations

Although the group format and structured content of each Seeking Safety group is similar, each group is profoundly distinct. Some have more mental health issues, differing cognitive levels, some are more dedicated to the group and recovery in general than others, some present as very angry while others are profoundly sad. This goes for individual members as well as the groups as a whole. There are commonalities also, not only in their shared experiences when actively using, but in members' dedication to confidentiality, which makes the group a safe place. Most groups have disclosed that confidentiality is an issue in all other groups, causing them to opt not to participate. The group members appreciate the self-determination we afford them, in allowing them to make up their own rules, starting where they are with the check-in every group and validating their experiences. The section on compassion usually has the most impact on the members, as it is for many the first time this concept of compassion for self was introduced to them. Members are also very responsive to exploring where their "harsh self-talk" comes from, and have expressed a desire to not teach their children to self-berate. Since many women have lost children in the system, this is a source of pain many women feel safe enough to explore in the group. It is often associated with strong feelings of guilt and/or defensiveness.

Many women do not have an internalized sense of safety. Therefore, it was found that putting the stage of "safety" in the context with other stages of recovery, "mourning" and "reconnection," was helpful. If the group is asked "why is it important to have safety before you begin to mourn?" the women can more easily process why safety is the first stage of recovery. All women know what mourning is, but most have a hard time defining safety.

Curriculum has differed slightly from group to group depending on the needs of particular members. Some chapters of Seeking Safety we have covered that were not in the original group format are: "Setting Boundaries," "Dealing with Anger," "The Life Choices Game" and "Healthy Relationships." Another chapter that we have more or less incorporated is the chapter on "Grounding." We found that once members begin to trigger a lot of feeling surrounding trauma, they need concrete ways to deal with their feelings when an individual counselor may not be available, such as if they wake from a nightmare at 3:00 in the morning. We routinely do grounding skills now with group members as well as give them examples of different grounding exercises they can refer to. Many of our members are often dissociated, and grounding is presented to them in this context as well. We may define dissociation for them, explain the dangers of being dissociated, i.e., on the street, but also normalize it as a common survival response to trauma and as a way of medicating their pain as always extremely profound. Often, women claim that they have attended many treatment programs but that they are only for the first time addressing their trauma in Seeking Safety.

There were times at the Dreitzer facility when women would not have child care during group time. If this obstacle could not be overcome by the group facilitators before the group, the children would have to attend group with the women. This only occurred a few times, but posed a dilemma for several reasons. The first was workable and could even be seen as a learning experience for members. Despite the children often being a distraction, the group leaders' interactions with them modeled appropriate ways to communicate and set limits with children. Facilitators also needed to explain to the members that we would not be able to get into deeper content when the children were present. However, this served to model appropriate boundaries for the members where their children were concerned. Facilitators were concerned about exposing the children to the traumatic content of the group and/or taking already limited intensive group time away. Members expressed the difficulty in associating their children with dark and oppressive pasts where they were abused, addicted, or traded sex for drugs. Early in their treatment and in the intervention, some women found the feelings that were triggered too overwhelming and were able to dissociate from them almost completely. The Dreitzer facility does offer frequent opportunities for individual therapy should anyone be in crisis, and facilitators always made themselves available after group. While monitoring the content, having the children in the group could actually give it a more intimate and safe feeling at times.

Administrative/System Observations

Therapeutic communities that provide comprehensive care are busy places and the larger the facility, the more difficult to maintain a feeling of safety. It just is not possible to establish the same kind of safety in a residential facility that one may be able to establish in a private therapist's office or outpatient clinic. Therefore, it is imperative that group leaders take extra measures to make their group time and space very safe and secure.

Vicarious traumatization and countertransference are a very significant piece of doing this work. Staff must receive the message from supervisors that it is acceptable to take care of themselves, and that symptoms of vicarious traumatization need to be normalized. Staff not educated about vicarious traumatization tend to minimize it or regard themselves as weak if they come across a story they have trouble hearing or being a witness to. Symptoms of vicarious traumatization including burnout may be ignored. Self-care needs should be promoted in order for successful trauma interventions with dually diagnosed clients to occur. Stigma about "receiving treatment" or going to "therapy" does not just exist among clients but among mental health and AOD staff as well. Just as alcohol and drug counselors have sponsors and continue to need to make meetings regularly, therapists need to feel entitled to seek out their own support systems.

The trauma-informed model of service differs from traditional groups found in AOD programs. The Portal Project departs from traditional treatment services and breaks through categorical, dichotomous thinking by thinking holistically about each woman. To simply label these women as addicts discounts some of the casual factors linking their personal histories, addiction, mental illness and traumatic experiences. The women in the study had the opportunity to celebrate themselves and actively participate in their recovery process. Specifically, the groups offer the women the opportunity to define and seek safety both internally and externally; to positively cope; and to connect with peers. Through the group process, the women began to understand the concept of safety when they first entered treatment. These groups also helped the women to look beyond labels to get a deeper understanding of their recovery process.

Crucial to the development of this gender-specific, layered approach to treatment is creating a receptive environment within the treatment center. Communication, collaboration and relationship are all important. Helping AOD staff to understand that this project was an addition to already existing services, not a replacement or substitute, lessened feelings that the project was a threat. Once built, the relationship supports numerous exchanges of information and transfer of skills and knowledge.

Another insight gleaned from this work has to do with the fact that client change is mirrored in the parallel process of systems change. The slow and often tentative regard for accepting the notion of change and managing ambiguities implicit in the process are present with both the client and the treatment setting as they seek out an integrated approach to care. By layering the model intervention to address key aspects of the problem, multiple opportunities to affect change are created. Relationship building, collaboration, cross-system planning and coordination promote the best thinking and strengthen bonds of teamwork. Finally, the importance of working with a supportive team throughout this process was essential. Working with an effective team enhances the work in support of women in recovery.

REFERENCES

Abbott, A. (1994). A Feminist Approach to Substance Abuse Treatment and Service Delivery. *Social Work in Health Care*, 19(3/4), 67-83.

Bollerud, K. (1990). A Model for the Treatment of Trauma-Related Syndromes Among Chemically Dependent Inpatient Women. *Journal of Substance Abuse Treatment*, 7, 83-87.

Brown, G., Anderson, B. (1991). Psychiatric Comorbidity in Adult Inpatients with More Than One Co-occurring Disorder. *American Journal of Psychiatry*, 148, 55-61.

Brown, V., Huba, Melchior, L. (1995). Level of Burden: Women with More Than One Co-Occurring Disorder. *Journal of Psychoactive Drugs*, 27(4) Oct-Dec.

Collins, J. J., Kroutil, L.A., Roland, E.J., Marlee-Guerra. (1997). Issues in the Linkage of Alcohol and Domestic Violence Services. *Recent Developments in Alcoholism*, 13, 387-405.

Finkelstein, N. (1994). Treatment Issues for Alcohol and Drug Dependent Pregnant and Parenting Women. *National Association of Social Workers*. 7-11.

Herman, J. L. (1992). *Trauma and Recovery*. New York: Basicbooks.

Kofed, L., Friedman, M.J., Peck, R. (1993). Alcoholism and Drug Abuse in Patients with PTSD. *Psychiatric Quarterly*, 64(2), 151-171.

Konrad, E.L. (1996). A Multi-Dimensional Framework for Conceptualizing Human Services in Integration Initiatives. *New Directions for Evaluation*, 5(19).

Substance Abuse and Mental Health Services Administration. (1998). *Cultural Competence Performance Measures for Managed Behavioral Healthcare Programs*.

New Directions for Families:
A Family-Oriented Intervention for Women Affected by Alcoholism and Other Drug Abuse, Mental Illness and Trauma

Nancy R. VanDeMark, MSW
Ellen Brown, PhD
Angela Bornemann, BS
Susan Williams, AA

SUMMARY. In conjunction with the SAMHSA-funded Women with Co-Occurring Disorders and Violence Study, Arapahoe House refined and evaluated an intervention integrating treatment for substance dependence, mental illness, and trauma for women and their dependent children. The New Directions for Families program combines comprehensive residential and outpatient treatment with parenting and self-sufficiency skills development. The program provides gender-specific, culturally sensitive, and strengths-oriented services for families in a two-phase program over eight months. Services include treatment for individual recovery in each of the three problem areas–mental health, alcohol and other drug abuse, trauma; basic needs of the family including employment; and social and family support systems. Consumers are in-

Nancy R. VanDeMark, Ellen Brown, Angela Bornemann, and Susan Williams are affiliated with Arapahoe House.

[Haworth co-indexing entry note]: "New Directions for Families: A Family-Oriented Intervention for Women Affected by Alcoholism and Other Drug Abuse, Mental Illness and Trauma." VanDeMark, Nancy R. et al. Co-published simultaneously in *Alcoholism Treatment Quarterly* (The Haworth Press, Inc.) Vol. 22, No. 3/4, 2004, pp. 141-160; and: *Responding to Physical and Sexual Abuse in Women with Alcohol and Other Drug and Mental Disorders: Program Building* (ed: Bonita M. Veysey, and Colleen Clark) The Haworth Press, Inc., 2004, pp. 141-160. Single or multiple copies of this article are available for a fee from The Haworth Document Delivery Service [1-800-HAWORTH, 9:00 a.m. - 5:00 p.m. (EST). E-mail address: docdelivery@haworthpress.com].

volved in all aspects of the project–in designing and implementing the intervention and evaluation and in governing the project through participation on the project's local and national steering committees.   *[Article copies available for a fee from The Haworth Document Delivery Service: 1-800-HAWORTH. E-mail address: <docdelivery@haworthpress.com> Website: <http://www.HaworthPress.com> © 2004 by The Haworth Press, Inc. All rights reserved.]*

KEYWORDS. Alcoholism, drug abuse, women, physical abuse, sexual abuse, children, residential

INTRODUCTION

My name is Sondra and I am a heroin addict. During the seven years I used heroin, I had attempted several times to stop using with no or little success. My family began to have very little to do with me, and I seemed to be constantly in and out of jail. Those years were horrific. When I look back it was a living hell. I was dying a slow physical death as well as an emotional and spiritual death.

–Sondra

Women seeking a stable position in our society encounter profound barriers when burdened with histories of incarceration, domestic violence, or AOD abuse, escalated by a context of growing stigma. Women troubled by multiple, simultaneous problems–including alcohol and other drug (AOD) dependence, trauma histories, and mental illness–face even greater challenges. In Colorado, the Arapahoe House *New Directions for Families* program has developed an intervention that responds to the complexity of these intersecting problems. Serving women with dependent children aged 12 and under, this family-oriented program integrates treatment for substance dependence, mental illness and trauma with the skills development required for long-term self-sufficiency and recovery.

STATEMENT OF THE PROBLEM

I began my career as an addict when I took my first drink at age nine. I loved the warm, funny feeling it gave me. I quickly made my way up the ladder of drugs. I took my first hit of crack when I was twenty-four. I found the escape I was looking for my whole life. I quickly became addicted and my habit was a very expensive one, not just monetarily, but in every aspect of my life. I used heavily with my husband for five years, then I became pregnant. I vowed never to touch the stuff again. Months later, my water broke while I was taking a hit. My daughter was born at just 4 pounds and positive for cocaine. It took her almost a minute to start breathing. Social Services were called and they took custody of my baby. My heart broke that day.

–Meg

Many studies highlight the relationship between violence, AOD problems and mental health disorders. Miller, Maguin, and Downs (1997), Downs and Miller (1998), and Hurley (1991) found an increased risk of psychiatric problems and alcohol abuse in adulthood associated with childhood physical and sexual victimization. Others confirm links between childhood abuse, Post Traumatic Stress Disorder (PTSD), and chemical dependence (Medrano, Zule, Hatch, & Desmond, 1999; Kunitz, Levy, McCloskey, & Gabriel, 1998; Bell, Duncan, Eilenberg, Fullilove, Hein, Innes, Mellman, & Panzer, 1994; Kilpatrick, Resnick, Saunders, & Best, 1998).

Need for Integrated, Gender-Specific, Culturally Appropriate Services

Many organizations independently treat one or more of the many problems faced by families affected by mental health, AOD problems, or trauma-related disorders, but services are often fragmented and difficult to access. Inadequate cross-disciplinary staff training, philosophical differences, cumbersome administrative structures, and insufficient funding complicate access to services (Ridgely & Dixon, 1993; Fazzone, Holton, & Reed, 1997; Grella, 1996; Minkoff, 1997). Interorganizational collaboration has been effective in addressing these problems with families (Fazzone et al., 1997; Finkelstein, Kennedy, Thomas, & Kearns, 1997; Melaville & Blank, 1991; Bell et al., 1994).

Research also indicates that AOD treatment programs serving women are more effective when designed specifically to account for their unique needs and their dependent children (Peterson, Gable, & Saldana, 1996). Gender-specific treatment for women should include comprehensive screening on physical abuse, sexual abuse and PTSD (Teets, 1995) and comprehensively address issues such as health, parenting, employment, and training in addition to treatment for AOD problems, mental health disorders and victimization (Finkelstein et al., 1997; Drabble, 1996; Liebschutz, Mulvey, & Samet, 1997). Because women often are the primary caregivers, treatment interventions are needed to mitigate the negative impact of a mother's AOD problems on her children. Miller, Smyth, and Mudar (1999) found that mothers with AOD abuse histories are more punitive with children, as are mothers with histories of partner and parental violence. A strong association exists between parental AOD problems and child abuse potential (Wolock & Magura, 1996; Miller et al., 1999), and AOD treatment settings offer an opportunity to intervene in these intergenerational concerns.

Involving women with personal recovery experience in the design and delivery of services offers an effective strategy for tailoring services to the family needs (Bell et al., 1994; Dixon, Cross, & Lehman, 1994; Prescott, 2000). The active involvement of women in the service delivery process has many benefits to recovery including contact with positive role models; specific skills development; improved self-esteem, recovery, and well-being; and decreased isolation and recidivism. Organizations benefit from improved quality of services and systems; reduced stigma; increased client engagement and retention for treatment and research; and enhanced research designs and interpretations of findings (Prescott, 2000).

HISTORY OF ARAPAHOE HOUSE AND NEW DIRECTIONS FOR FAMILIES

Arapahoe House is a community-based nonprofit organization committed to the provision of accessible, affordable, and effective services for individuals and families with alcohol, drug, and other behavioral health problems. Arapahoe House has provided AOD services since 1976 and is now Colorado's largest alcohol and drug treatment agency, serving over 16,000 unduplicated clients annually in 15 locations across the metro Denver area.

The Arapahoe House *New Directions for Families (NDF)* program began in 1995 with funding from the Center for Substance Abuse Treatment (CSAT) within the Substance Abuse and Mental Health Services Administration (SAMHSA). Initiated as a residential AOD treatment center for women and children, the facility provides comprehensive services for families. In 1998, Arapahoe House became a study site for the SAMHSA-sponsored Women with Co-Occurring Disorders and Violence Study to develop and evaluate integrated services for women affected by substance abuse, mental illness and trauma. NDF became the site of the experimental intervention for this study, enhancing the availability of on-site mental health services and adding trauma-specific services to provide an integrated intervention.

TARGET POPULATION

Table 1 characterizes clients entering NDF from 1/1/01 to 2/15/02 as part of WCDVS. Clients all had substance dependence, mental health disorders, and trauma histories, nearly half were Caucasian, with an average age of 29, and one-third "never married."

INTERVENTION PHILOSOPHY AND PHASES

Philosophy

Basic to New Directions for Families (NDF) is the belief that family-oriented, integrated treatment services for women with substance dependence, mental health disorders, and trauma are more effective than a sequential service approach. Building on this premise, NDF incorporates several complementary approaches in its treatment philosophy to maximize effectiveness: (a) The Stages of Change Model; (b) Motivational Interviewing; (c) Cognitive-Behavioral Approach; (d) Solution-Focused Approach; and (e) Integrated Services for Substance Dependence, Mental Illness, and Trauma. Each of these approaches is delivered in the context of a family-oriented setting that emphasizes both the enhancement of the parent-child relationship and the woman's individual recovery. As a therapeutic model, the approaches powerfully effect positive change in families whose mothers have AOD problems, psychiatric disorders, and histories of violence.

Stages of Change Model and Motivational Interviewing. NDF incorporates tenets of the Stages of Change model (Prochaska & DiClemente, 1982; Prochaska, DiClemente, & Norcross, 1992), which holds that people change behaviors by progressing through five stages: pre-contemplation, contemplation, preparation, action, maintenance. Motivational interviewing is a non-authoritative technique for helping people to comprehend their own motivations and resources and resolve their ambivalence about

TABLE 1

Women Entering New Direction for Families from 1/1/01 to 2/15/02 (n = 57)	
CHARACTERISTIC	*PERCENT or MEAN*
Average Age	29 years
Current Substance Dependence	100 %
Current Axis I Disorder:	
Mood Disorders	75%
Anxiety Disorders	40%
Other Axis I	7%
Axis II Disorder	19%
Lifetime Trauma History:	
Emotional Abuse	68%
Physical Abuse	86%
Sexual Abuse	58%
Substance of Choice:	
Cocaine	30%
Methamphetamine/Stimulants	23%
Alcohol	16%
Marijuana	12%
Opiates	11%
Dual addiction/Polydrug	9%
Race/Ethnicity:	
Caucasian	49%
Hispanic	30%
African American	21%
American Indian	12%
Other	4%
Marital Status:	
Never married	33%
With a significant other/partner	30%
Divorced/Separated	21%
Currently married	16%
Children:	
Mean number of children per family	2.55
Mean number of children per family served at NDF	1.23
Mean age of children served	3.45

changing. The technique is persuasive rather than coercive, and supportive rather than argumentative.

Cognitive-Behavioral Approach. The NDF staff use cognitive and behavioral techniques to help the clients identify the thoughts and assumptions they have developed in reaction to traumatic experiences in their past and examine the impact these have had on their behavior, including their addictions (see Corsini & Wedding, 1989). Cognitive therapy uses behavioral techniques to modify automatic thoughts and assumptions. The process involves experimenting with different behaviors and bringing into question specific maladaptive beliefs; the result can be new learning. The counselor helps the client identify errors in thinking and maladaptive assumptions, exploring how these patterns of thinking have impacted her life.

Solution-Focused Approach. Elements of Solution-Focused therapy (Berg & Miller, 1992) reflect the NDF philosophy that clients have many strengths and should be empowered and involved in their treatment. Healthy activities and past successes are emphasized, as are clients' strengths, frames of reference, and mutual cooperation between client and counselor. This collaborative approach highlights the active involvement of clients in treatment.

Integrated Services for Substance Dependence, Mental Illness, and Trauma. Attention to issues related to mental illness, AOD problems and trauma are fully integrated into all support and therapeutic activities. NDF staff believe that these issues are interrelated and must be addressed together. The program incorporates the interrelation of problems in these ways:

- Basic education about physical, sexual, and emotional abuse and witnessed violence must address how current behaviors including AOD abuse are linked to past abuses. Re-framing current symptoms as clients attempt to cope with unbearable trauma is necessary as well for individual recovery to be lasting.
- An essential part of treatment is the development of basic skills in self-regulation, boundary maintenance, communication, the development of healthy relationships, female sexuality, and correcting distorted thoughts and beliefs.
- Trauma-informed education about healthy parenting and life skills for children will help ensure children's healthy psychological development.
- The treatment environment should be safe and supportive in order to provide the basis for addressing painful and difficult treatment issues.

Many of the critical service components of trauma-specific intervention are the same as those of AOD and/or mental health treatment. Consequently, the gains women make in trauma-related groups often translate to a positive effect on treatment in the other two areas as well.

The Phases of the Intervention

Phase I. The NDF program consists of three phases extending over approximately eight months. During the first few months, Phase I focuses on three main areas: (a) intensive treatment for AOD problems and mental health disorders, (b) treatment related to current or past trauma, (c) parenting skills based on an individualized treatment plan. Individual and group therapies develop skills for abstinence and mental health, coping with lasting effects of trauma, and improving parenting. Education addresses family health, safety, and basic life skills. Phase I also includes comprehensive evaluation of the family, psychiatric evaluation and necessary treatment, and case-management linkage to services such as medical care, children's mental health treatment, cultural development and support, recreation, and recovery groups. Once firmly grounded in their recovery effort and parenting skills, women may advance to Phase II.

Phase II. Phase II emphasizes three primary areas: employment skills, job placement, relapse prevention. The program employs a vocational specialist to assist the woman in developing skills aimed at immediate employment/education and self-sufficiency. Women work full time or participate in unpaid employment in conjunction with job training. Women also prepare for the transition into the community by locating appropriate housing, enrolling their children in childcare or school, and developing a relapse prevention plan. During this time, women are encouraged to be active in peer support groups inside and outside the facility.

Phase III. Supporting the gains made in residential treatment, Phase III begins when a woman returns to the community, usually after four months of residential treatment at NDF. This continuing care phase of treatment includes a continuing care treatment group; linkage with services in the community; and an alumni group providing social support.

> I enjoy coming to continue care, it really helps in my recovery. I have learned to set boundaries and I have a whole new life. I've completely changed my routines, and my life has more structure.
>
> –Kathy

Phase III also includes POWER (Power of Women Recovery)–the Alumni Program that provides social support for the families currently in residential treatment as well as those who are now residing in the community. POWER conducts a formal meeting once a month and occasional fundraising activities to support the expenses associated with their plans. This group also plans and implements individual support and recreational activities for women and for families, both providing support for recovery and reinforcing family health.

INTERVENTION SERVICES

Skills and Resource Development

Throughout each of the three phases of NDF programming, services are oriented to developing skills and resources in the three areas of *individual recovery, basic needs of the family including employment,* and *social and family support systems.* These areas develop at different rates for different women and their families, and success in one area may co-exist with relapse in another. Each woman's resources and resiliency determine how she progresses in each of these areas. When she can balance all three without relapse, she achieves self-sufficiency.

I. Individual Recovery. Individual recovery encompasses the internal process of recovery from substance dependence, mental illness, and trauma. This process includes building self-esteem and meaning in life. Individual recovery issues are addressed through individual and group counseling, education, cultural activities, skills development, communication, assertiveness, decision making, problem solving, spirituality, journaling, using positive daily affirmations, drawing or creative writing, meditating, and practicing positive communication skills. The program also attempts to model the larger community. Women are expected to exercise skills necessary to live in the community, such as learning to compromise, giving and receiving support, establishing boundaries, and upholding individual responsibility.

Treatment activities supporting individual recovery include those services aimed specifically at AOD problems, mental illness, and trauma and those that integrate attention to all three disorders and how they impact parenting. Individual and group education and counseling sessions address each of these categories of activity. Mental health and trauma treatment activities complement the addiction treatment process. Mental health and AOD problems are viewed through a trauma-informed lens. The consulting psychiatrist and community mental health centers provide medication management for symptomatic concerns. In individual and group therapy modalities, women use explorative and reflective techniques to uncover the developmental and historical roots of their mental health and trauma issues and cognitive-behavioral techniques to manage symptoms in daily functioning.

> Certain set times, familiar places, and regular activities associated with drinking have been woven closely into the fabric of my life. Like fatigue, hunger, loneliness, anger, and over escalation, these old routines can prove to be traps and dangerous to our sobriety. When I first stopped drinking, I found it useful to look back at the habits surrounding my drinking and whenever possible to change a lot of the small things connected with drinking.

> –Kathy

Individual Recovery: AOD Services. Individual and group therapy use an integrated stages of change approach, addressing drug and alcohol effects, withdrawal and consequences, maternal AOD abuse, HIV and infectious illnesses, relapse prevention, the impact of AOD problems on families, developing substance-free support systems, and leisure skills. During the first phase of treatment, women receive AOD treatment six days a week for about two hours a day and thereafter, 2-3 times a week in two-hour sessions. Women attend on- and off-site, peer-run support groups, including Alcoholics Anonymous, Narcotics Anonymous, Cocaine Anonymous, and Women in Recovery, three times a week.

Individual Recovery: Services for Mental Health Disorders. Psychiatric evaluation and treatment, individual counseling, and education on mental illness and psychotropic medication address mental health disorders. Treatment services are provided about two times a week for 6-8 hours during the first few months of treatment and approximately weekly thereafter. The local mental health center or the Arapahoe House psychiatric consultant provides psychiatric evaluation and oversees pharmacological treatment.

Individual Recovery: Trauma-Specific Services. These services are aimed at two discrete problems: childhood victimization and domestic violence. Women are assessed for the extent and nature of their trauma history and are never coerced to address trauma issues. Instead they are provided with information and given choices about participation in individual and group trauma activities. NDF adapted for a residential treatment setting the 24-session outpatient Trauma Recovery and Empowerment Model (TREM) designed to address issues of sexual, physical and emotional abuse (Harris & The Community Connections

Trauma Work Group, 1998). Phase I of TREM addresses gender identity, sexuality, interpersonal boundaries, and self-esteem. Phase II of TREM covers sexual, physical, and emotional abuse, specifically the interaction of the abuse with mental health issues, AOD problems and relationships. The first 16 sessions of TREM occur in partially open groups meeting twice a week. The aim is to have women complete these sessions before they enter the Reintegration Phase (NDF Phase II). The Phase II trauma group is held once a week in the evening and covers sessions 17-24. The self-help workbook, *Healing the Trauma of Abuse* (Copeland & Harris, 2000), orients women to the trauma material before they enter the group. Using the self-help workbook, women can enter the group in sessions #4, #6, and #9 of the TREM curriculum after having individually completed the sessions already covered in group. The self-help workbook is also used for women who are not ready to address their trauma issues in the group but who would like to participate in individual trauma treatment.

> It was very hard for me to face my issues of abuse and trauma. The TREM program helped me see clearly what I had been through and gave me a safe haven to cope with everything. I learned many skills to deal with my pain and how to avoid such things in the future.

> –Meg

Trauma-specific services for domestic violence include safety planning, linkage with legal assistance, and individual and group counseling. Clients spend two-to-four hours a week in group therapy for the first two to three months at NDF with program staff trained in trauma recovery for the dually diagnosed. The group is modeled on the book *Journey Beyond Abuse: A Step by Step Guide to Facilitating Women's Domestic Abuse Groups* (Fischer & McGrane, 1997). The group covers the definition of domestic abuse, patterns and types of abuse, and the cycle of violence, abusive relationships, anger shame and guilt, self-care, and healthy relationships. Women gain insight into why they have developed certain destructive behaviors and relationships and learn tools to create healthier lives for themselves and their children.

Individual Recovery: Services That Address Recovery from All Three Problems. As mentioned earlier, attention to issues of mental illness, AOD problems and trauma are integrated throughout the program. Skills development activities integrate all three areas and include assertiveness, communication, self-esteem, anger management, personal empowerment, spirituality, cultural development, relationships, safety, self-care, and symptom management.

II. Basic Needs. Basic life skills in wellness, health, nutrition, stress management and financial planning are integral components of the NDF program and are incorporated into all phases. Groups focus on the following topics weekly: HIV risk reduction, STD prevention, maternal AOD abuse, violence, nutrition, child health, budgeting, and financial issues. Additionally, women conduct daily stress management activities such as morning meditation and stretches. Financial planning begins at the moment a woman enters the program, as she starts allocating finances to savings and spending accounts and makes good-faith payments on her outstanding debts, including treatment costs incurred.

> New Directions helped me put together a resume and get a great job, they gave me many relapse prevention tools, evaluated my mental health and treated me for depression, my husband and I got some marriage counseling sessions, and I even learned how to cook.
>
> –Meg

Basic Needs: Employment and Vocational Services. NDF staff or community organizations provide a full range of employment and vocational services, including a complete assessment of work history; related strengths and barriers; GED tutoring and testing; and computerized occupational job search and job skills tutorials. Individual and group sessions aim to improve job acquisition and retention skills. Interagency agreements with local TANF, Vocational Rehabilitation offices, and community colleges also provide a wealth of resources.

Women at NDF are required to work full time in paid employment or engage in a combination of unpaid work and training for at least 30 days prior to successful discharge from the residential setting. During this time, women make arrangements for peers to take their children to the Child Learning Center or school bus stop. Women must prepare meals and care for their children. Additionally, evening treatment activities target relapse prevention, family strengthening, trauma-related issues, and community reintegration. The responsibility to balance attention to individual recovery issues, work, and parenting mirrors the experience women will face upon transition back into the community. During this time, staff and peers provide support and assistance with problem solving to prepare women and children for the transition.

Basic Needs: Housing. Locating safe and affordable housing is a monumental issue for women in transition. Upon admission to NDF, women learn about housing subsidies and options, and most women are placed on waiting lists for Section 8 vouchers. Even with subsidies, the search for appropriate housing located near employment, childcare, and social support systems can be very difficult. Women with felony convictions face an added burden of locating landlords who are willing to take a chance on their integrity.

Basic Needs: Transportation. Another challenging aspect of reintegration is transportation. During the residential stay, van service, bus tokens, and cab vouchers are available to transport women to some outside commitments. But upon leaving the program, women must find their own transportation and balance this difficulty with the other challenges faced during transition.

Basic Skills: Childcare. Children from the age of infancy through pre-school attend the licensed Child Learning Center at NDF, a therapeutic educational environment that includes three classrooms organized by children's age. An early childhood educator supervises the classroom, implementing weekly lesson plans based on thematic units. Activities enhance science, art, math, literature and gross motor skills. Prior to leaving the program, women are referred to the Colorado Child Care Assistance Program for cash assistance with childcare, while the Child Learning Center staff assist women in selecting a childcare center. Learning to balance the demands of the most basic needs such as childcare, job, housing, and transportation while also developing resources for individual recovery teaches clients the importance of building strong social support systems as they travel toward self-sufficiency.

III. Social and Family Support. Women entering NDF usually have minimal social support. Often, friends and family are current alcoholics or drug abusers. The women have severed relationships with those who do not abuse substances; or family and friends who do not abuse have severed relations with the women because of abusing behaviors. Many women have been engaged in romantic relationships that were abusive or not supportive. Learning to develop healthy support systems is essential for the journey toward self-sufficiency.

Social and Family Support: Family Services. NDF's comprehensive family services begin with a Family Therapist's assessment of each family, including familial composition, strengths, cultural and spiritual relationships, disciplinary practices and issues, sources of support, and current issues, and development of individualized treatment goals. The Family Therapist attempts to engage the women's non-abusive partners and extended families in treatment to learn about addiction, family dynamics, and healthy communication. The multi-family group meets 1 to

1.5 hours weekly and teaches women how to be effective in providing healthy support systems for the recovery process. Clients are encouraged to have their significant others attend with them, as it provides an opportunity to gain a better understanding of the struggles that clients have endured and will likely face during recovery.

Social and Family Support: Parenting Services. NDF stresses activities that build parenting skills with a trauma-informed perspective and reflect constructive and educational discipline. Positive reinforcement, limit-setting, and reasonable, reinforceable consequences are commonly used to promote healthy, loving family time. Corporal punishment is prohibited during the family's residential stay and discouraged as a disciplinary technique. Women are encouraged to learn new, more effective techniques of parenting and are allowed experiential support in implementing these new ideas. Mothers learn a variety of behavioral modification techniques that respect and enhance self-esteem and teach children to make positive choices. The greatest parenting achievements experienced by women in this program are in building relationships with their children, developing patience, and creating quality family time. Basic to the NDF program is the realization that a lack of effective, positive parenting skills and an inability to deal with children's problems can contribute to relapse after discharge. An interfamily parenting group, based on the *Nurturing Program for Families in Substance Abuse Treatment and Recovery* modified for residential AOD settings (Moore, Buchan, Finkelstein, & Thomas, 1997), is provided to women and their children during the course of their stay at NDF. The eight-session curriculum covers the core domains of appropriate developmental expectations: developing empathy, alternatives to corporal punishment, and child-parent role reversal. Parenting groups, interfamily groups, and multi-family groups each meet for 1 to 1.5 hours a week. In addition, each family has the opportunity to meet with the Family Therapist for a weekly one-on-one session, allowing the therapist to address each family's clinical needs individually.

Social and Family Support: Children's Services. Using a family-oriented approach, NDF addresses the preventive and treatment needs of the children both directly and indirectly. The multi-family group and the interfamily group indirectly enhance the child's well-being and development by building extended families into support systems. Services have also been developed that directly address trauma-related experiences encountered by children and mental health issues that stem from their mother's substance use and mental illness. (Another article in this issue details the services provided through the Children's Subset Study.)

Consumer/Survivor/Recovering Person (CSR) Integration

Over the years of the study, Arapahoe House has involved women (known as CSRs) with personal experience in recovery from the effects of AOD problems, mental illness and trauma (known as consumer/survivor/recovering persons or CSRs). These individuals assist the professionally credentialed staff at NDF in understanding the needs of women and providing suggestions for improving services. The mission of consumer integration in the program has been improvement of the quality, accessibility and responsiveness of services for women and children through meaningful involvement of individuals with personal recovery experience throughout the program and its management. Clients are viewed as full partners in identifying their goals for treatment plans, and clinical staff assist them by suggesting interventions that are likely to result in goal attainment. The consumer integration effort has consisted of several elements: (a) employment of recovering persons as staff members and participants in the agency steering committee managing the grant, (b) a continuing care treatment group co-facilitated by CSRs, (c) an alumni group providing social support, (d) qualitative exit interviews with women leaving treatment, and (e) frequent focus groups conducted to provide feedback on improvement of services.

A CSR Liaison staff position facilitates coordination of all consumer activities with the larger program services and advocates for consumer issues with the larger organization. The CSR liaison also facilitates relapse prevention and parenting groups and participates in agency and community committees. A Peer Case Manager helps link clients with services, assists in acquiring transportation, and advocates with external resources for client benefit. The case manager position is responsible for conducting an assessment of ancillary service needs, preparing treatment plans, and facilitating a case management group aimed at improving access to community services. A primary aspect of the peer case manager's role is transporting, advocating and supporting the clients with outside appointments such as court appearances, doctor's appointments and housing. While both positions provide support, advocacy and continuity of care, they also serve as role models for clients. These positions also aid staff with monitoring the milieu, mediating conflict between clients, and co-facilitating groups such as TREM and the children's intervention group. The CSR positions receive monthly scheduled supervision both individually and in a group and may access a supervisor for daily difficulties. The CSR staff positions have also been an integral part of the monthly meetings of the steering committee overseeing the design, implementation, and evaluation of the intervention; one or both positions have also represented consumer concerns at the cross-site National Steering Committee meetings held several times annually.

The consumer liaison and peer case manager also coordinate the alumni support and advisory body entitled POWER (Power of Women Engaging Recovery). This group (a) assists in the facilitation of the Continuing Care group; (b) reviews program materials, schedules, and policies to ensure they are consumer friendly; (c) organizes social support activities; and (d) coordinates the consumer involvement in local and national committees. Consumers participating in the project are compensated for time spent consulting with the program; however, they agree that an important motivation for participation in the alumni group is that "service work" is part of their recovery. POWER meets weekly and is supported organizationally with access to computers, transportation, Internet, and a telephone as needed to perform duties. Consumers are involved with state and community committees, bringing women's voices to legislative and other entities that can influence change to services provided to this population. Furthermore, exit interviews and focus groups conducted throughout the life of the study have provided feedback used by NDF staff to improve services.

> New Direction has a strong CSR group, which I have been able to utilize as well as giving back to the community. I believe that if I stay connected to the women at New Directions my chance of remaining clean and sober will increase.
>
> –Kathy

LESSONS LEARNED

Arapahoe House staff have learned a number of lessons about the difficulties and benefits of juggling funding, integrating CSRs, and delivering integrated services to women affected by AOD problems, mental illness, and trauma.

Modeling Healthy Lifestyles

Modeling healthy lifestyles may be one of the most important roles of residential treatment staff. For individuals who have spent a lifetime in chaotic and often violent substance-abusing homes, experiencing a safe, structured environment can instill hopefulness for recovery. For NDF staff, consumer representatives, and alumni, demonstrating how to balance the demands of parenting with maintaining personal recovery goals and financially supporting a family appears to be critical for women who have never experienced this balance in their own childhood.

Providing Services for Children

The literature has demonstrated the significant negative impact that a mother's AOD problems, mental illness, and history of victimization has on her children. Through the course of development of the program, the need to provide therapeutic services for children has emerged as a priority need among the families served. The project staff have recognized the need to conduct a comprehensive assessment and link clients with a broad set of community resources in order to meet the complex needs–both preventive interventions and rehabilitative services–of children whose mothers enter the program. Promoting relationships with other adults to include other parents and extended family can be a challenging yet essential part of implementing a services plan for children. Employing nurturing men on the staff to serve as positive role models for children is crucial.

Attending to Transitions

Through the qualitative study and consumer discussions, the importance of support and resources in the face of transitions has emerged. The common transitions are recognized to be when a woman first becomes employed or loses her employment, when school or training programs commence, and when the family moves from residential treatment to community-based treatment. NDF graduates cite this transition back into the community as the most stressful event in their treatment experience. Change is stressful for anyone; women in early recovery as well as their children are particularly vulnerable to periods of transition. Women are often subject to stigma and discrimination as a result of their illnesses, social status, gender, and culture. Preparing women to overcome these experiences may assist them to avert a relapse to job loss, substance use, or mental illness. For these reasons, NDF has implemented a variety of supports to help families develop skills of compromise and conflict resolution to ease the difficult transition out of residential services and into the community. The supports found to be most helpful include: (a) structured peer support groups such as POWER and Continuing Care groups, (b) job retention skills, (c) assertive linkage with community resources while a family is in residential treatment, (d) childcare and transportation assistance, and (e) peer case management aimed specifically at the transition from residential treatment to the community.

Working with the Larger Community

Treatment of families with complex problems does not happen in a vacuum. Staff at programs helping families with multiple problems must be knowledgeable of agency and community resources. Programs must respond to local, state, and federal policy changes that affect eligibility for social programs and changes in public perception. From the point of referral for services, staff must include all agencies involved in the life of the family. Child welfare and probation agencies often have very specific and sometimes court-ordered expectations for the family. Child custody orders and the wishes and concerns of non-custodial parents must be respected. Staff in these programs must be able to understand the distinct goals of agencies such as child welfare, probation and parole, and TANF offices, and to assist the women to develop a plan that satisfies all of these goals and requirements. Program staff must be attentive to involving community groups, including spiritual and cultural supports, in the treatment program. Staff must assist families to use cultural and spiritual strengths to support recovery.

Involving Consumers in All Aspects of the Treatment Program

Involvement of consumers in the development and implementation of the integrated treatment program at NDF has resulted in numerous benefits. The value of the partnership between consumers and staff begins in the development of the treatment plan. Consumers who are meaningfully involved in the development of their own treatment plans are more likely to have an active investment in their treatment and to feel empowered to meet the challenges of recovery. The POWER group members carry out this goal of empowerment as they arrange community activities such as garage sales benefiting clients, the Women's Recovery Day celebration, Christmas and New Year's parties for residential clients, publication of the POWER newsletter, focus groups, and policy and procedure changes within Arapahoe House.

In summary, staff have discovered that assisting families with multiple problems to overcome obstacles requires an active partnership between program and family characterized by mutual respect, a comprehensive view of the challenges, and a vision of a healthy future.

We cannot keep what was freely given to us if we do not give back to others who may be struggling. My life today is beautiful. I wake up next to a wonderful child and I can take care of her without being hung-over or dope sick. I struggle financially but make ends meet with the help of resources that I learned about at New Directions. I have my family back in my life today and those people thought that I was hopeless. Today I love myself and other people do too. In the 12-step program we learn of the promises that will materialize for us if we work a simple program. I am here to tell you it's true!

–Sondra

REFERENCES

Bell, R., Duncan, M., Eilenberg, J., Fullilove, M., Hein, D., Innes, L., Mellman, L., & Panzer, P. (1994). *Violence against women in the United States: A comprehensive background paper.* New York: The Commonwealth Fund.

Berg, I. & Miller, S. (1992). *Working with the problem drinker: A solution focused approach.* New York: W. W. Norton.

Copeland, M.E. & Harris, M. (2000). *Healing the trauma of abuse: A women's workbook.* Oakland, CA: New Harbinger.

Corsini, R.J. & Wedding, D. (1989). *Current psychotherapies* (4th ed.). Itasca, IL: F.E. Peacock.

Dixon, L., Krauss, N., & Lehman, A. (1994). Consumers as service providers: The promise and challenge. *Community Mental Health Journal, 30*(6), 615-625.

Downs, W.R. & Miller, B.A. (1998). Relationships between experiences of parental violence during childhood and women's self-esteem. *Violence and Victims, 13*(1), 63-77.

Drabble, L. (1996). Elements of effective services for women in recovery: Implications for clinicians and program supervisors. *Chemical dependency: Women at risk* (pp. 1-21). NY: Harrington Park.

Fazzone, P., Holton, J., & Reed, B. (1997). *Substance abuse treatment and domestic violence.* Rockville, MD: Center for Substance Abuse Treatment. Treatment Improvement Protocol (TIP) Series 25.

Finkelstein, N., Kennedy, C., Thomas, K., & Kearns, M. (1997). *Gender specific substance abuse treatment.* Center for Substance Abuse Prevention, Contract No: 277-94-3009.

Fischer, K.L. & McGrane, M. (1997). *Journey beyond abuse: A step by step guide to facilitating women's domestic abuse groups.* Amherst H. Wilder Foundation.

Grella, C. (1996). Background and overview of mental health and substance abuse treatment systems: meeting the needs of women who are pregnant or parenting. *Journal of Psychoactive Drugs, 28*(4), 319-343.

Harris, M. & The Community Connections Trauma Work Group. (1998). *Trauma recovery and empowerment: A clinician's guide for working with women in groups.* New York: Free Press.

Hurley, D. (1991). Women, alcohol, and incest: An analysis review. *Journal on Studies on Alcohol, 52*(3), 253-268.

Kilpatrick, D.G., Resnick, H.S., Saunders, B.E., & Best, C.L. (1998). Victimization, posttraumatic stress disorder, and substance use and abuse among women. In C.L. Wetherington & A.B. Roman (Eds.), *Drug addiction research and the health of women* (pp. 285-307). Rockville, MD: National Institute on Drug Abuse, U.S. Department of Health and Human Services.

Kunitz, S.J., Levy, J.E., McCloskey, J., & Gabriel, K.R. (1998). Alcohol dependence and domestic violence as sequelae of abuse and conduct disorder in childhood. *Child Abuse and Neglect, 22*(11), 1079-1091.

Liebschutz, J.M., Mulvey, K.P., & Samet, J.H. (1997). Victimization among substance-abusing women: Worse health outcomes. *Archives of Internal Medicine, 157*, 1093-1097.

Medrano, M.A., Zule, W.A., Hatch, J., & Desmond, D.P. (1999). Prevalence of childhood trauma in a community sample of substance-abusing women. *American Journal of Drug and Alcohol Abuse, 25*(3), 449-462.

Melaville, A. & Blank, M. (1991). *What it takes: Structuring interagency partnerships to connect children and families with comprehensive services.* Washington, DC: Education and Human Services Consortium.

Miller, B.A., Maguin, E., & Downs, W.R. (1997). Alcohol, drugs and violence in children's lives. In M. Galanter (Ed.), *Recent developments in alcoholism: Vol. 13. Alcohol and violence* (pp. 357-385). New York: Plenum Press.

Miller, B.A., Smyth, N.J., & Mudar, P.J. (1999). Mothers' alcohol and other drug problems and their punitiveness toward their children. *Journal of Studies of Alcohol, 60*(5), 632-642.

Minkoff, K. (1997). Integration of addiction and psychiatric services. In K. Minkoff & D. Pollock (Eds.), *Managed mental health care in the public sector: A survival manual* (pp. 233-245). The Netherlands: Harwood Academic Publishers.

Moore, J., Buchan, B., Finkelstein, N., & Thomas, K. (1997). *Nurturing program for families in substance abuse treatment and recovery.* Park City, UT: Family Development Resources.

Peterson, L., Gable, S., & Saldana, L. (1996). Treatment of maternal addiction to prevent child abuse and neglect. *Addictive Behaviors, 21*(6), 789-801.

Prescott, L. (2000). *Consumer/survivor/recovering women: A guide for new partners in collaboration.* Women, Co-Occurring Disorders and Violence Coordinating Center, Policy Research Associates. Delmar, NY. January Draft.

Prochaska, J.O. & DiClemente, C.C. (1982). Transtheoretical therapy: Toward a more integrative model of change. *Psychotherapy: Theory, Research, and Practice, 19*, 276-288.

Prochaska, J.O., DiClemente, C.C., & Norcross, J.C. (1992). In search of how people change: Applications to addictive behaviors. *American Psychologist, 47*, 1102-1114.

Ridgely, M.S. & Dixon, L.B. (1993). *Integrating mental health and substance abuse services for homeless people with co-occurring mental and substance use disorders.* Center for Mental Health Services of the Substance Abuse and Mental Health Services Administration of the U.S. Department of Health and Human Services.

Teets, J.M. (1995). Childhood sexual trauma of chemically dependent women. *Journal of Psychoactive Drugs, 27*(3), 231-238.

Wolock, I. & Magura, S. (1996). Parental substance abuse as a predictor of child maltreatment re-reports. *Child Abuse & Neglect, 20*(12), 1183-1193.

Allies:
Integrating Women's Alcohol, Drug, Mental Health and Trauma Treatment in a County System

Jennifer P. Heckman, PhD
Frances A. Hutchins, MPA
Jennifer C. Thom, MA
Lisa A. Russell, PhD

SUMMARY. Allies, one of nine sites participating in the Substance Abuse Mental Health Services Administration's Women, Co-occurring Disorders and Violence Study, was developed through collaboration between California's San Joaquin County Health Care Services and ETR Associates. Allies was charged with developing and implementing integrated services for women with ADM disorders and abuse histories within the County. Stakeholders identified service enhancements that were implemented in alcohol and drug treatment programs: integrated case management, trauma groups, and integrated parenting classes. Approximately 400 providers attended training activities; 174 women par-

Jennifer P. Heckman is affiliated with ETR Associates. Frances A. Hutchins is affiliated with San Joaquin County Office of Substance Abuse. Jennifer C. Thom and Lisa A. Russell are affiliated with ETR Associates.

[Haworth co-indexing entry note]: "Allies: Integrating Women's Alcohol, Drug, Mental Health and Trauma Treatment in a County System." Heckman, Jennifer P. et al. Co-published simultaneously in *Alcoholism Treatment Quarterly* (The Haworth Press, Inc.) Vol. 22, No. 3/4, 2004, pp. 161-180; and: *Responding to Physical and Sexual Abuse in Women with Alcohol and Other Drug and Mental Disorders: Program Building* (ed: Bonita M. Veysey, and Colleen Clark) The Haworth Press, Inc., 2004, pp. 161-180. Single or multiple copies of this article are available for a fee from The Haworth Document Delivery Service [1-800-HAWORTH, 9:00 a.m. - 5:00 p.m. (EST). E-mail address: docdelivery@haworthpress.com].

161

ticipated. Allies experienced barriers and successes. Lessons learned may be useful for future change efforts. *[Article copies available for a fee from The Haworth Document Delivery Service: 1-800-HAWORTH. E-mail address: <docdelivery@haworthpress.com> Website: <http://www.HaworthPress. com> © 2004 by The Haworth Press, Inc. All rights reserved.]*

KEYWORDS. Alcoholism, drug abuse, women, physical abuse, sexual abuse, children, integration

INTRODUCTION

Allies, one of nine sites participating in SAMHSA's Women, Co-occurring Disorders and Violence Study (WCDVS), was developed through collaboration between San Joaquin County Health Care Services (HCS) and ETR Associates in Northern California. This project's purpose was, with meaningful consumer involvement, to develop, implement, and evaluate comprehensive, integrated, trauma-informed and trauma-specific services for women with alcohol/other drug use and mental disorders and physical and/or sexual abuse histories. In addition, in collaboration with three of the other eight SAMHSA sites, this project was charged with implementing an intervention for children, ages 5-10, of the women participating in the larger women's project.

The primary goals of the women's project were to reduce the women's alcohol and drug use and mental health and trauma-related symptoms and improve their parenting abilities. Goals for the children's project were comparable: to prevent or reduce the intergenerational perpetuation of violence, alcohol and drug abuse, and mental health problems, as well as the impact of violence on children. The overall project was divided into two phases: the planning, development, and early implementation occurred in the first two years (Phase I) with full implementation and outcome and process evaluations occurring in the final three years (Phase II). Below is a description of the background, development and implementation of the women's intervention,[1] including lessons learned that may assist others in developing integrated services for this population.

THE PROBLEM

The consequences of interpersonal trauma can include the development of post-traumatic stress disorder (PTSD), other mental health disorders, and alcohol and/or other drug abuse. Traditional mental health, alcohol and other drug (AOD), and trauma treatment approach these issues as distinct and separate disorders rather than recognizing the cyclical and etiological connections between these issues and the detrimental impact of this connection on a woman's life. Further, women with co-occurring alcohol/other drug and mental health disorders and trauma have tended to receive poor prognoses and been considered difficult to treat and lacking in motivation (U.S. Department of Health and Human Services, 2000). Yet Brown (1997) and Grella (1996) argue that the problem frequently lies not within the women, but rather within the disparate systems of care and service delivery.

Accessing traditional care systems requires women personally to coordinate their care across independent systems with variant philosophies, approaches, and goals (Grella, 1996), a burden that would be minimized with more integrated care. Harris (1994, 1996) and Najavits, Weiss, Shaw, and Muenz (1998) demonstrate that integrated treatment approaches are appropriate for women with ADM disorders, and Brown (1997) points out that these approaches treat women more holistically by synthesizing philosophies and eliminating conflicting messages. Ultimately, coordinated services and integrated treatment philosophies, at both the systems and client levels, alleviate some of the challenges confronting the individual seeking treatment (Brown, 1997), with flexible services, allowing for individual choice, frequently resulting in the most success (National Institute on Drug Abuse, 1999).

THE ENVIRONMENTAL CONTEXT

Allies was implemented for women with ADM disorders and trauma that were receiving county-run services in San Joaquin County, a rapidly growing semi-urban county in Northern California. Stockton, San Joaquin's County seat, has a highly diverse population and is the urban center for several rural agricultural communities. As the County center, Stockton served as the primary location of this service integration effort. San Joaquin County HCS collaborated with ETR Associates, a not-for-profit health education, training, and research organization, to develop, implement and evaluate Allies so as to better serve the needs of this project's target population in their community.

THE TASK

Allies' primary goals were to reduce women's alcohol and drug abuse and their mental health and trauma-related symptoms, as well as increase their parenting abilities. A further goal was to meaningfully include consumer/survivor/recovering women (CSRs) (i.e., women from the target population) in all aspects of the project to ensure the most culturally appropriate and effective services as possible.

Allies was specifically charged with developing integrated treatment strategies that required both client- and system-level change efforts. At the cross-site level, the national Steering Committee required eight key intervention components for client-level service delivery: (1) outreach and engagement; (2) screening and assessment; (3) treatment activities; (4) parenting skill development; (5) resource coordination and advocacy; (6) trauma-specific services; (7) crisis intervention; and (8) peer-run services. The premise behind the individual-level change effort was to incorporate existing resources into this more comprehensive and integrated new service delivery system to the extent possible. After a careful review of existing services within San Joaquin County, Allies staff determined that three new client-level intervention components were required: trauma-specific services; resource coordination and advocacy (to be accomplished through integrated case management); and integrated parenting skills development. On the system-level, mental health and alcohol and other drug providers needed to become more trauma-informed.

TARGET POPULATION

The target population consisted of women, 18 years and older, with ADM disorders and physical and/or sexual abuse histories. Specific eligibility criteria required that women have DSM-IV Axis I and/or II disorders and have experienced two or more AOD or mental health treatment episodes during their lifetimes (with one currently active and the other active within the prior five years). The 176 women participating in this project ranged in age from 19 to 60 years (mean age = 37.2 years). Of these women, 81.0% were referred from AOD treatment, 9.2% were self-referred, 8.6% were referred from mental health services, and 1.1% were referred from trauma treatment providers.

THE INTERVENTION'S DEVELOPMENT

The Phase I systems- and client-level interventions were developed with the involvement of, and input and guidance from, stakeholders throughout the community. Within the first month of funding, Allies' three direct service staff were hired and the Allies Coordinating Council (ACC) was formed. The Allies staff represented the three integrating agencies (the Office of Substance Abuse [OSA], Mental Health Services [MHS], and the Women's Center, a local non-profit trauma service agency) and two out of three of these women were CSRs. Drawing staff that represented both the target population and the agencies targeted for integration proved vital to inter-agency buy-in and began to set the stage for integration. The ACC served as the project's local Steering Committee in the first year of planning and included AOD, mental health, and trauma treatment providers and again, in many instances, CSRs. This Council met monthly and provided an important mechanism for enhancing integration and cooperation among service providers. The ACC provided an opportunity to learn more about each service provider's philosophy and approaches to treatment, and, ultimately, quite importantly served as a vehicle to get to know one another that resulted in far-reaching favorable impacts throughout the duration of the project.

After one year it was determined that the ACC, while tremendously successful in bringing professionals and paraprofessionals together to discuss the target population's needs, was too large (with 30 participants) to accomplish the detailed planning and development needed. A structural change was then implemented: the ACC joined forces with an existing Dual Diagnosis Task Force to continue their discussions and the Core Providers Board was created. This new Board included two representatives from each of the three disciplines (mental health, AOD, and trauma) and Allies team members; the Board met monthly through the end of Phase I to guide and finalize the Phase II implementation design.

A CSR Advisory Board was also formed in Phase I that continued into Phase II. This Board facilitated the active engagement of target population members in the design of both the intervention and its evaluation.

Systems-Level Intervention Development

The goal of the system-level development work was to increase provider awareness of the needs and benefits of effectively collaborating across disciplines for the well-being of their mutual clients. Community-wide strategies for accomplishing this goal included presentations, newsletters, pamphlets, and posters on the importance of integrated, trauma-informed, and trauma-specific services for the target population. Allies also provided large training events (see Figure 1)[2] that were complemented by County-provided trainings in areas such as dual diagnosis and pharmacology and diversity in the workplace. CSRs participated in all of these events.

Individual-Level Intervention Development

A Phase I Allies local needs assessment identified specific service gaps for this population within San Joaquin County.[3] Resulting recommendations included the need for trauma-specific services for the ADM population; greater integration across mental health, alcohol and drug abuse, and trauma treatment; and trauma- and ADM-informed parenting classes. The needs assessment results also indicated that coordinated care, in addition to benefiting the individual consumer, would benefit the community at large by significantly reducing inappropriate referrals and ineffective treatment modalities, and their resulting negative impact on the system (Crews, Hutchins, & Heckman, 2000).

Based on the needs assessment, input from the national cross-site Steering Committee, a literature review and extensive discussions with and guidance from the project's Boards, Allies staff identified the models and curricula that would be used for addressing these unmet community needs.

Trauma-Specific Services. Allies staff identified and presented to local stakeholders published interventions designed to address women's trauma recovery, taking into account the particular needs of the commu-

FIGURE 1. Allies Phase I Community Cross-Discipline Provider Training Events

Training Topic Area	Total Participants
Relapse Prevention	68
Domestic Violence	18
Dual Diagnosis and PTSD	69
Seeking Safety and Assessing PTSD	87
Trauma Recovery Empowerment Model (TREM)	122
Strengths-based Case Management	80
Nurturing Parenting	94

nity. Selection criteria for the trauma intervention encompassed three major issues. First, the varying length of San Joaquin treatment programs favored short-term (less than 90 day) interventions. Secondly, there was concern among AOD treatment providers that addressing PTSD with women new to recovery could result in severe relapse. County providers were familiar and comfortable with a sequential treatment approach in which a period of abstinence is required before trauma issues are addressed. Thirdly, the backgrounds of those who would provide the intervention were considered. Those identified as most likely to provide the trauma groups consisted of a variety of paraprofessional and professional staff with varying levels of training, many of whom were CSRs with their own trauma histories. Therefore, selecting a model that could be provided by paraprofessionals, as well as highly trained clinical professionals, was seen as preferable.

Herman's (1992) Trauma and Recovery Model, used as the foundation for many trauma-specific interventions, was favored by many stakeholders. This model views trauma recovery as occurring over three stages: (1) the need to establish safety; (2) remembrance and mourning; and (3) reconnection. Two specific group interventions, drawing in part from Herman's model, emerged as the most promising based on their theoretical underpinnings and empirical evidence of effectiveness: Seeking Safety (Najavits, Weiss, Shaw, & Muenz, 1998; Najavits, 2002) and the Trauma and Recovery Empowerment Model (TREM) (Harris, 1996; Harris & Community Connection Trauma Work Group, 1998). Both Seeking Safety and TREM assist women in examining the role of AOD and mental health disorders in their lives and how these issues relate to traumatic life events (Harris, 1996; Najavits, Weiss, Shaw, & Muenz, 1998). Both also assume that survivors recover in stages, from establishing safety to reconnection with others (Herman, 1992; Lebowitz, Harvey, & Herman, 1993).

Seeking Safety focuses primarily on the first stage of trauma recovery and is based on the premise that alcohol and other drug use is a coping mechanism for managing severe PTSD symptoms. Seeking Safety provides a context where women learn and practice safe coping skills as alternatives to alcohol and other drug use. TREM, on the other hand, addresses all three stages of recovery.

Allies sponsored training sessions on both curricula so that stakeholders and staff would be thoroughly informed when choosing between the two. These trainings were well attended and discussions of both interventions were later facilitated. Seeking Safety was favored for early trauma work because it allayed the fear of some stakeholders that the trauma intervention would be too overwhelming for women early in recovery. Seeking Safety had the additional advantage of being a curriculum that could be facilitated by the paraprofessional counselors in the County's AOD treatment settings. The notion that clients could later be referred to TREM groups, facilitated by professional mental health providers, for more in-depth trauma work was viewed as an ideal option for accommodating the size of the affected population with the existing provider mix.

It was ultimately decided that Seeking Safety would be offered as the first step for women in their trauma recovery, with TREM offered as a later stage treatment. It was also decided that Seeking Safety, a 24-week curriculum, would be divided into two 12-week series with the first series open (allowing women to join at any time) and the second closed (to allow greater trust levels to develop). Splitting the curriculum in this way would allow women, particularly those in 3-month treatment programs, to experience success through their completion of the first series; all women would then have the option and be encouraged to participate in the second Seeking Safety series. TREM, a 33-week curriculum, would be provided for those women interested in committing to deeper work. In preparation for implementation, Allies contracted with the curriculum developers to conduct training sessions on both curricula for alcohol and drug counselors and mental health clinicians. To maintain fidelity to the models, the project also established ongoing clinical supervision for those providing these services.

Service Coordination. Case management's role in the intervention model was debated among stakeholders. Some viewed case management as the stabilizing factor for all clients and, although Seeking Safety included a group case management component, that additional individual case management was critical for truly integrating services and assisting clients in accomplishing their goals. Yet other stakeholders were concerned that adding individualized case management would result in service duplication because many clients would be receiving service coordination from their existing alcohol and drug and mental health providers. Ultimately, it was decided that Allies would offer multiple case management levels. With this model, participants would have the option of choosing the mode of case management that best met their needs (e.g., no case management, service coordination from an existing provider, Seeking Safety group case management, intensive individual case management from Allies staff, or a combination of more than one option). The initiation, length, and intensity of services would be determined by client preference.

Several case management models have demonstrated effectiveness for persons with chronic mentally illness, yet few have been tested with those in alcohol and drug treatment. However, Rapp's (1992) strengths-based case management model, while originally developed for work with persons with mental illness, was successfully adapted for assisting people with AOD problems (Goldstein, 1997; Rapp, Siegal, & Fisher, 1992; Rapp, personal communication, May 2, 2000; Weick & Chamberlain, 1997). This model focuses on individual strengths over pathology, assumes that every consumer has unlimited growth potential, views the consumer as the director of her treatment, and seeks resources from the community (Saleeby, 1997). Strengths-based case management also has been demonstrated to increase treatment retention, reduce relapse rates, and improve resource acquisition (Rapp, Harvey, & Fisher, 1992). Rapp's strengths-based case management (SB-CM) model was ultimately selected for the intervention's resource coordination component because it was conceptually aligned with Allies' philosophy of the need to empower women (i.e., to allow them their "voice") and because of its demonstrated success for individuals with AOD issues.

The University of Kansas, School of Social Work had conducted extensive research and training on Rapp's model. In preparation for implementation, Allies contracted with the University of Kansas to provide community service provider training on SB-CM. After the training, the project made minor adaptations to the model to better reflect the population to be served and the County's environmental conditions.

Integrated Parenting Curriculum. The national cross-site Steering Committee charged each of the projects with identifying and implementing a parenting curriculum that would address the specific needs of mothers with ADM disorders and trauma histories. However, finding a parenting curriculum that met these requirements proved a formidable task. After an extensive literature search, Allies staff identified the Nurturing Program for Parents (Bavolek & Comstock, 1983) and Nurturing Families Affected by Substance Abuse, Mental Illness, and Trauma (Institute for Health and Recovery, 2001) as the most suitable. While stakeholders liked the Nurturing Programs, they required that the parenting curriculum match both the length of most County alcohol and drug treatment programs and met local Child Protective Services requirements. Neither of these curricula met both of these requirements. The decision ultimately was made to develop an adapted curriculum blending Nurturing Program for Parents and Children Birth to Five Years (Bavolek & Dellinger-Bavolek, 1985), Nurturing Families Affected by Substance Abuse, Mental Illness and Trauma (Institute for Health and Recovery, 2001), and the existing San Joaquin County OSA parenting curriculum.

Based on these three curricula and with input and guidance from parenting instructors and other community providers, project staff and the CSR Advisory Board developed the 12-week Recovering Families curriculum. Recovering Families was designed to blend discussions and activities around parenting issues particular to the target population with sessions focusing on specific parenting skills. This curriculum, approved by the Child Welfare Unit Chief of Child Protective Services, was piloted in the community prior to full implementation and was well received by both the participants and the parenting instructors.

ROLE OF CONSUMER/SURVIVOR/RECOVERING WOMEN (CSRs)

Meaningfully involving women from the target population in the development and implementation of the intervention, as well as its evaluation, was central to this project's design (SAMHSA, 1998). Based on the conviction that life experience provides the potential for invaluable contributions to planning, decision making, and service provision, CSRs were actively involved in all aspects of the Allies project. In Phase I, CSRs worked as Allies staff and ACC members and later as members of the CSR Advisory and Core Provider Boards. While a primary Phase I role for Allies CSR staff members was to provide client services, these staff also participated actively in CSR volunteer recruitment, Board activities, needs assessment focus groups, and in national cross-site Steering Committee meetings. Through this work emerged the undisputed need for coordinated care and integrated treatment for women with ADM and trauma histories. Each of these activities was driven by the intent to develop intervention services and an evaluation design that reflected and was sensitive to the needs of the target population.

During Phase I, CSRs also contributed considerably to evaluation design issues such as recruitment and retention, peer support for women participating in research interviews, tracking, incentives, potential barriers, and data collection and measurement. CSRs also provided community outreach and education activities, including implementing a Trauma Anonymous group, developing guidelines for CSR volunteer positions, laying the groundwork for a video documentary, and participating on CSR panels that generated greater community awareness. All of these activities resulted in significant CSR contributions to the final client-level intervention model and the evaluation design.

In Phase II, with much of the planning and development complete, Allies CSR staff placed the vast majority of their emphasis on providing client services through their work as case managers and Seeking Safety group facilitators. Based on CSR recommendations, the evaluation team hired CSRs to provide peer support for women as they went through the interviewing process. These staff also assisted in tracking clients for research interviews and in discussions of the preliminary results of the study. Non-CSR evaluation staff supported CSR contributions to the evaluation by providing short workshops on research fundamentals and ongoing support.

Volunteer CSR contributions also continued into Phase II. Advisory Board activities included refining the parenting curriculum and developing both a community CSR resource packet and a newsletter for sharing information on community resources, helping others to understand what it means to be a CSR, and inspiring hope. Further, a group of Phase I clients (and their prior group facilitator) formed the NEW (Newly Enlightened Women) group to continue their Seeking Safety work into Phase II and practice leadership skills. During the first year and a half of Phase II, the Advisory group continued to meet monthly and the NEW group met weekly; halfway through Phase II both groups came to a close due to struggles to find meaningful missions.

THE INTERVENTION'S IMPLEMENTATION

Phase II implementation benefited significantly from an additional Phase I outcome that occurred in conjunction with the intervention's development. As a result of the Phase I training, ACC and Board members contributions, and Allies staff activities, a substantial increase in community awareness of the needs of women with ADM disorders and trauma histories was realized. Allies, and its goals, had become well known and appreciated throughout the treatment community, setting the stage for the intervention's implementation.

Systems-Level Implementation

With the planning stage behind and implementation ahead, the Core Provider Board disbanded and was replaced with the implementation-focused Primary Treatment Network (PTN) Board to assist in launching and overseeing implementation. The PTN Board was comprised of the three AOD treatment program directors who supported the implementation of Allies at their five sites, Allies' Intervention Director, Allies' Principal Investigator and a Research Associate involved in the process evaluation data collection. The PTN Board met formally three times (approximately quarterly) during the implementation start-up phase to review and discuss the treatment interventions and the support needed from their staffs. Various additional issues (e.g., eligibility requirements, concerns regarding the sensitive issues raised in the baseline interviews, evaluation activities) were discussed. After the first year of Phase II, the Board did not continue to meet formally. However, the Intervention Director worked individually with PTN directors to provide guidance, answer questions, discuss challenges, and brainstorm solutions. Also in Phase II, the Dual Diagnosis Task Force, having been in existence for 10 years in San Joaquin County, continued to meet monthly. The Task Force's mission, as a result of Allies Phase I, was now broadened to include discussions of the needs of women with ADM disorders *and* trauma histories.

Individual-Level Implementation

The Primary Treatment Network (PTN), the primary Phase II implementation sites, consisted of five alcohol and drug programs that served either women only or had large proportions of women. Allies' grant-funded staff consisted of an Intervention Director for the women's and children's projects (80% and 10% time, respectively),[4] a lead clinical case manager (50% time), and two CSR AOD counselors/case managers (each at 100% time). The cross-site evaluation design required a substantial sample. The targeted minimum sample size was 137 women to study over a 12-month period and, because attrition was expected, Allies staff were encouraged to engage even larger numbers of women in services. Effectively providing the intervention for such large numbers of women, by the limited numbers of staff members supported by the grant, was daunting.

As discussed, the primary client-level service enhancements designed in Phase I for Phase II implementation were trauma-specific groups (i.e., Seeking Safety, to be followed by TREM), SB-CM, and the Recovering Families parenting curriculum. Allies direct service staff (the three case managers) were to facilitate the trauma-specific groups[5] and provide SB-CM for clients; OSA parenting instructors would implement the new integrated parenting curriculum. Due to resource limitations and philosophical constraints, two Phase II changes to this intended service enhancement model occurred. TREM, piloted in Phase I with some OSA staff members, was not implemented during the study's evaluation of the intervention. Throughout the study intervention period, Allies staff intended to begin TREM groups; however, due to time limitations, a TREM group did not begin until data collection was essentially complete.[6] Similarly, SB-CM also was not implemented due to time restrictions, but also to philosophical challenges in implementing this model. PTN paraprofessional counselors *and* Allies case managers experienced SB-CM as time consuming and many counselors experienced it as mismatched with their training; counselors were accustomed to developing treatment plans that were problem/needs-focused, rather than strengths-focused. These two issues were ultimately insurmountable and SB-CM was abandoned with "intensive integrated case management" taking its place. Giving up SB-CM, a model with demonstrated success for individuals with alcohol and drug issues, was a disappointment. However, the primary intent of the intervention's "resource coordination and advocacy" component was to support participants in receiving integrated AOD, mental health, and trauma treatment; the integrity of this focus remained throughout the intervention's implementation.

The implementation of the Phase II service enhancements (i.e., Seeking Safety, intensive integrated case management, and Recovering Families) is described below.

Seeking Safety and Integrated Case Management Implementation. Seeking Safety and integrated case management were new services to the community necessitating changes in philosophies and increased staff time. The Phase I design designated the Allies staff as primarily responsible for the implementation of these intervention components, but the numbers of women needing services were large, and the number of Allies staff available to provide Seeking Safety and case management was very limited. Several strategies were designed to address this disparity. First, Allies planned to use a "trainer of trainers" model whereby Allies case managers would facilitate Seeking Safety groups with an on-site treatment program counselor as a co-facilitator. A clear advantage to this model was that each group (of ideally eight to 12 women), would have two facilitators; but the potentially even greater advantage was that the co-facilitators would become experienced Seeking Safety leaders and able to facilitate their own groups. By engaging counselors as Seeking Safety leaders, Allies case managers' time would be freed to provide more individualized intensive case management.

A second Phase II strategy for maximizing Allies case manager time was to house the two Allies CSR case managers at PTN sites, rather than at the off-site Allies office, thus creating greater client accessibility. With this model, the case managers were further positioned to promote trauma-informed, integrated services for the women in these programs. The lead case manager, still housed at the Allies office, provided Seeking Safety groups and intensive case management (when needed) for women without access to PTN services, as well as at one of the treatment programs.

During the first year and a half of Phase II, Allies contracted with a licensed clinician to provide biweekly clinical supervision for Allies staff to support Seeking Safety and case management implementation. As the project progressed (approximately nine months after implementation began), Allies contracted with a second clinician to provide clinical supervision, on a weekly or biweekly basis (depending on the treatment site) for all PTN counselors to assist them in providing integrated case management. This clinical supervision also provided opportunities for counselors to work through interpersonal conflicts and, quite importantly, to address countertransference issues that arose in their work with clients.

A further strategy for supporting the delivery of Seeking Safety groups and intensive case management was prompted by the resignation of an Allies CSR case manager. Due to the inability to fill this position, because of a County hiring freeze, ETR Associates, the lead agency on the grant and the project's evaluation "arm," contracted with two licensed clinicians to assist Allies staff in providing Seeking Safety and individual case management. These services were provided at the ETR office and at the program that had housed the case manager who had left the project. Because the ETR office was located less centrally than the other service sites, ETR peer support staff began providing transportation, when needed, for women to and from services.

Recovering Families Implementation. Over the first year of implementation, two OSA parenting instructors provided Recovering Families classes within the PTN. Frequently, the parenting instructors participated as advocates for the women in their classes by writing letters and conferencing with Children's Protective Services. The parenting instructors reported that the curriculum prompted "breakthroughs" where parents saw the ways that they were continuing the abuse cycles and actively looked for ways to stop those cycles. At approximately mid-point in the implementation phase (after the OSA receipt of additional funding to provide more widespread parenting classes), five additional parenting instructors were recruited to provide Recovering Families within the PTN and at other community treatment sites.

ACHIEVEMENTS, CHALLENGES, LESSONS LEARNED

Allies' implementation successes, challenges encountered, and lessons learned are presented below. These points may be useful to others embarking on similar missions.

Launching a Cross-Discipline Service Integration Change Effort

Allies' implementation required that providers: expand their treatment philosophies; work with clients in new ways; increase their collaboration; and maximize available resources. Involving cross-agency providers as Allies staff proved vital to inter-agency buy-in and set the stage for integration. Further, Phase I broad stakeholder involvement (primarily through the ACC, Core Providers and CSR Boards), the extensive cross-discipline provider training, and the community needs assessment resulted both in community recognition of this change effort and in a community-needs focused implementation plan. Yet significantly altering service delivery philosophies and approaches across large numbers of providers requires time. Allies had two years to accomplish these vital foundations; more time may have resulted in broader changes.

> *Lesson 1.* Involve staff in key roles from the agencies that you want to integrate.
> *Lesson 2.* Involve a broad array of stakeholders in planning and development.
> *Lesson 3.* Provide stakeholders with extensive training and opportunities for discussion and relationship building.
> *Lesson 4.* Know that planning and development take time and allow for it.

Consumer Involvement

The breadth of knowledge brought by CSRs to Allies, much gained through life experience, resulted in culturally sensitive approaches for addressing women's needs that would not have occurred without their involvement. Project CSR staff crossed the formal educational spectrum from those lacking a high school diploma (or GED) to those with master's degrees; several staff had considerable alcohol and drug counselor work experience while others, more recent in their recovery, had minimal job experience. With the assistance of other staff, those with less work experience developed skills that greatly benefited the project as well as enhanced their capabilities for productive work in other settings. With the invaluable contributions of these women also came challenges: two staff members relapsed; some experienced boundary and/or dual relationship issues with clients; some found aspects of their work re-traumatizing; and some struggled with desired skill sets. Further, volunteer CSRs, while interested in making ongoing Phase II contributions, lacked sufficient non-consumer staff leadership and support (due to their engagement in other project activities) for facilitating these contributions.

> *Lesson 5.* Involve target population members in all aspects of the change effort.
> *Lesson 6.* Provide target population staff and volunteers with the support, training, and leadership needed for their success.
> *Lesson 7.* Train non-consumer staff in approaches for supporting their consumer colleagues.

Service Provider Training and Support

The extensive Phase I training of Allies, PTN, and additional OSA and MHS staff increased provider knowledge of both the needs of and approaches for better serving the target population. Further, the Phase II Allies and PTN staff clinical supervision provided ongoing opportunities for skill development. These training mechanisms strengthened and broadened the provider base of those who could effectively deliver Seeking Safety and integrated case management services. Yet staff turnover resulted in service delivery interruptions and compromised the Seeking Safety "train-the-trainer" model's success, with fewer PTN staff facilitating trauma groups than had been hoped. Finally, because of the trauma histories of many PTN staff, service delivery frequently raised challenging personal issues and dissuaded some from wanting to facilitate trauma services.

> *Lesson 8.* Expect staff turnover and provide ongoing training and support accordingly.

Lesson 9. When target population members are involved in service delivery, recognize that countertransference issues may arise and support may be needed.

Client Engagement in Services

Qualitative evaluation data reflected that many women viewed Allies' service enhancements as positively impacting their healing and recovery, yet service participation was less than expected. While empowering women to make their own treatment choices was intrinsic to Allies, non-mandatory service participation resulted in a lack of receipt of consistent services for many women. Partially successful strategies for supporting participation included staff calls to women to remind them of their upcoming groups or individual sessions and, later, when many women needed transportation to and from the less centrally located "service enhancement" site, to both coordinate and provide the transportation. However, providing transportation across the PTN was not feasible, and reminder phone calls, while helpful, did not ensure that women would show up for their services. Women inconsistently participated or dropped out for various reasons: childcare and transportation issues, as well as personal crises, were common; and, for women further along in their recovery, busy work or school lives made participation less of a priority. Further, it was observed that for many women a "window of opportunity" existed to engage them in services; e.g., if a woman indicated her interest in services but had to come back later to get started, the opportunity for service engagement might have been lost. Finally, psychological treatment readiness, particularly for trauma work, undoubtedly affected participation levels, as did living lives where struggles to meet basic needs (e.g., housing, food) were of higher priority than service participation.[7]

Lesson 10. Know the treatment barriers (e.g., transportation, childcare) your population faces.

Lesson 11. Provide external client supports (e.g., reminder phone calls, transportation, childcare) for increasing service participation when resources permit.

Lesson 12. When possible, engage women in services immediately following their expressed interest.

Lesson 13. Client treatment readiness (influenced by external as well as psychological factors) will strongly influence service participation.

Resource Limitations

Rarely, if ever, are resources as bountiful as would be desired in large-scale change efforts. Additional resources across all aspects of this change effort would have benefited the target population greatly. As indicated, this change effort likely would have benefited from more time for planning and development, but additional, and critical, other resource limitations existed. Three direct service staff were the only providers whose primarily responsibilities were to implement Allies' services–a severe limitation when so many women needed to be served. Further, many women were interested in and may well have benefited from psychotherapy, yet due to insufficient funding and inadequate insurance reimbursements, few Allies women were able to receive these services. Finally, community resource limitations at large had profound impacts on these predominantly low-income women. For example, wait lists of two to eight years existed for subsidized housing and rental vacancy rates were very low, with the costs of rentals continuing to rise over the duration of this project's implementation.

> *Lesson 14.* Develop realistic goals keeping in mind resource constraints.
> *Lesson 15.* Be as creative as possible in maximizing all existing resources.

CONCLUSIONS

Profound challenges exist in large change efforts: resistance to change naturally occurs; expected and unexpected barriers arise; efforts to address challenges may or may not be successful. Despite planning processes' sophistication, not everything goes as hoped. Allies' development and implementation were not exceptions to these axioms inherent in change efforts. Yet Allies' achievements, over a relatively short period, must not be underestimated. Significant change occurred, women's lives were positively impacted, and much was learned.

NOTES

1. See Finkelstein et al. (in press) for a complete description of the children's cross-site intervention.
2. Out of a pool of approximately 750 providers, 395 providers participated in at least one of Allies' training events.

3. The needs assessment data were based on nine CSR focus groups, seven staff focus groups, and 11 individual interviews with lead administrators throughout the County.

4. A year into Phase II, an Assistant Director, both a CSR and prior drug counselor, was hired at 80% time across both projects and the Intervention Director reduced her time to 35% across both projects.

5. The lead case manager, a clinician, was intended to facilitate the TREM groups in addition to Seeking Safety.

6. Because of TREM's late implementation, the effectiveness of this model in San Joaquin was not evaluated.

7. While case management services, in addition to efforts to coordinate mental health, alcohol and drug treatment, and trauma services, were intended to assist clients in attaining basic needs such as shelter, community resources were limited and such case manager efforts were not always successful.

REFERENCES

Bavolek, S.J. & Comstock, C.C. (1983). *Nurturing Program for Parents and Children 4-12 Years.* Park City, Utah: Family Development Resources, Inc.

Bavolek, S.J. & Dellinger-Bavolek, J. (1985). *Nurturing Program for Parents and Children Birth-5 Years.* Park City, Utah: Family Development Resources, Inc.

Brown, V. (1997). *Breaking the Silence: Violence/Abuse Issues for Women Diagnosed with Serious Mental Illness.* Culver City, CA: Prototypes Systems Change Center.

Crews, J., Hutchins, F., & Heckman, J. (2000). *San Joaquin County Needs Assessment: Women Survivors of abuse with co-occurring substance abuse and mental health disorders.* Unpublished manuscript.

Finkelstein, N. et al. (in press). Building resilience in children of mothers who have co-occurring disorders and histories of violence: Intervention model and implementation issues. *Journal of Behavioral Health Services and Research.*

Goldstein, H. (1997). Victims or victors? In D. Saleeby (Ed.), *The Strengths Perspective in Social Work Practice.* White Plains, New York: Longman.

Grella, C. (1996). Background and overview of mental health and substance abuse treatment systems: Meeting the needs of women who are pregnant or parenting. *Journal of Psychoactive Drugs, 28,* 319-343.

Harris, M. (1994). Modifications in services delivery and clinical treatment for women with severe mental illness who are also survivors of sexual abuse trauma. *Journal of Mental Health Administration, 21,* 397-406.

Harris, M. (1996). Treating sexual abuse trauma with dually diagnosed women. *Community Mental Health Journal, 32,* 371-385.

Harris, M. & Community Connection Trauma Work Group. (1998). *Trauma Recovery and Empowerment.* New York, NY: The Free Press.

Herman, J.L. (1992). *Trauma and Recovery.* New York, NY: Basic Books.

Institute for Health and Recovery. (2001). *Nurturing Families Affected by Substance Abuse, Mental Illness and Trauma.* Cambridge, MA: Institute for Health and Recovery.

Lebowitz, L., Harvey, M.R., & Herman, J.L. (1993). A stage-by-dimension model of recovery from sexual trauma. *Journal of Interpersonal Violence, 8,* 378-391.

Najavits, L.M. (2002). *Seeking Safety: A Treatment Manual for PTSD and Substance Abuse.* New York, NY: The Guilford Press.

Najavits, L., Weiss, R., Shaw, S., & Muenz, L. (1998). Seeking Safety: Outcome of a new cognitive-behavioral psychotherapy for women with post-traumatic stress disorder and substance dependence. *Journal of Traumatic Stress*, 11, 437-456.

National Institute on Drug Abuse. (1999). *Principles of Drug Addiction Treatment: A Research-Based Guide.* (NIH Publication No. 99-4180). Rockville, MD: National Institutes of Health.

Rapp, R.C., Siegal, H.A., & Fisher, J. (1992). A Strengths-Based Model of Case Management/Advocacy: Adapting a Mental Health Model to Practice Works with Persons Who Have Substance Abuse Problems. In *Progress and Issues in Case Management.* National Institute on Drug Abuse Research Monograph 127.

Saleeby, D. (1997). The strengths approach to practice. In D. Saleeby (Ed.), *The Strengths Perspective in Social Work Practice.* White Plains, New York: Longman.

Substance Abuse Mental Health Services Administration, Public Health Service, Department of Health and Human Services, *Cooperative Agreement to Study Women with Alcohol, Drug Abuse & Mental Health (ADM) Disorders Who Have Histories of Violence, Guidance for Applicants* (GFA) No. TI 98-004, March 1998.

U.S. Department of Health and Human Services, Public Health Service, Substance Abuse and Mental Health Services Administration. (2000). *Substance Abuse Treatment for Persons with Child Abuse and Neglect Issues: Treatment Improvement Protocol (TIP) Series, 36* (DHHS Publication No. SMA 00-3357).

Weick, A. & Chamberlain, R. (1997). Putting problems in their place: Further explorations of the strengths perspective. In D. Saleeby (Ed.), *The Strengths Perspective in Social Work Practice.* White Plains, New York: Longman.

Integrated Trauma Services Teams for Women Survivors with Alcohol and Other Drug Problems and Co-Occurring Mental Disorders

Roger D. Fallot, PhD
Maxine Harris, PhD

SUMMARY. Integrated Trauma Services Teams (ITSTs) provide a model for addressing simultaneously and in a closely coordinated way the needs of many women survivors for trauma, AOD, and mental health services. Based on the principles of the Trauma Recovery and Empowerment Model (TREM) and centered on the TREM group intervention, these teams offer a trauma-informed context for integrated service delivery and emphasize the development and enhancement of specific trauma recovery skills. Drawing on the importance of gender and culture in understanding and responding to the concerns of women survivors, ITSTs feature individualized recovery plans, a range of trauma-informed group interventions, and peer supports. *[Article copies available for a fee from The Haworth Document Delivery Service: 1-800-HAWORTH. E-mail address: <docdelivery@haworthpress.com> Website: <http://www.HaworthPress.com> © 2004 by The Haworth Press, Inc. All rights reserved.]*

Roger D. Fallot and Maxine Harris are affiliated with Community Connections.

[Haworth co-indexing entry note]: "Integrated Trauma Services Teams for Women Survivors with Alcohol and Other Drug Problems and Co-Occuring Mental Disorders." Fallot, Roger D., and Maxine Harris. Co-published simultaneously in *Alcoholism Treatment Quarterly* (The Haworth Press, Inc.) Vol. 22, No. 3/4, 2004, pp. 181-199; and: *Responding to Physical and Sexual Abuse in Women with Alcohol and Other Drug and Mental Disorders: Program Building* (ed: Bonita M. Veysey, and Colleen Clark) The Haworth Press, Inc., 2004, pp. 181-199. Single or multiple copies of this article are available for a fee from The Haworth Document Delivery Service [1-800-HAWORTH, 9:00 a.m. - 5:00 p.m. (EST). E-mail address: docdelivery@haworthpress.com].

KEYWORDS. Alcoholism, drug abuse, women, physical abuse, sexual abuse, urban, integration

INTRODUCTION

The District of Columbia Trauma Collaboration Study (DCTCS) is a two-phase project addressing the needs of women trauma survivors with co-occurring mental health and substance use disorders. In Phase I, we conducted a process evaluation examining the perceived needs of, and services available for, women in the target population. We met with focus groups and interviewed consumers, clinicians and administrators in a number of alcohol and other drug (AOD) treatment and mental health service settings. In addition, project meetings and gatherings involving over 50 city agencies discussed clinical and systems obstacles to effective services and proposed innovative solutions. At the end of Phase I, we implemented in two agencies a package of trauma-informed, comprehensive, integrated services offered by Integrated Trauma Services Teams (ITSTs). The Trauma Recovery and Empowerment Model (TREM) approach, developed at Community Connections (the lead agency) over the past decade, provided the guiding principles as well as the primary clinical intervention, a 33-session manualized group for women survivors. Phase II of the project examined the effectiveness of this intervention by comparing it to "services as usual" care in similar agencies in another city. This paper describes the setting, background, and rationale for the development of ITSTs as well as the core components of this integrated approach to trauma, alcohol and other drug abuse, and mental health problems.

STATEMENT OF THE PROBLEM

The DCTCS addresses a broad range of interconnected problems related to trauma, mental health, and AOD abuse among women with histories of violent victimization. Our clinical experience, review of the literature, and the results of our Phase I process evaluation confirm that consumer/survivor/recovering persons (CSRs) need service programs that do the following:

1. Offer trauma-specific and trauma-informed services. Our systems assessment found a dearth of both *trauma-specific* and *trauma-informed* services in D.C. By *trauma-specific*, we mean services whose primary goal is to address the impact of abuse and other traumatic experiences and to facilitate trauma recovery. Other human services, not designed to address trauma directly, may be *trauma-informed* (Harris & Fallot, 2001). That is, policies, procedures and services reflect an understanding of key trauma-related psychosocial realities; services are offered in a way that reinforces basic elements necessary to trauma recovery; and their services do not retraumatize or revictimize CSRs. All services in the DCTCS, then, were designed and implemented in the context of a trauma-informed systems model.

2. Integrate mental health, AOD, and trauma services. The need for integrated services is not restricted to a small group of women. In our D.C. settings, over 70% of women with mental disorders have a co-occurring problem with the abuse of alcohol and/or other drugs, and virtually all of the women with co-occurring disorders have a history of trauma. We take as a fundamental assumption that integration of services occurs at both the clinical and the systems level. At the *clinical* level, integration means that different services addressing different problems are coordinated as closely as possible to ensure that interventions are continuous, compatible, and, whenever possible, simultaneous. Both CSR and provider focus groups in Phase I repeatedly highlighted the ways in which unrecognized or untreated mental health problems exacerbate substance use and vice versa. Discussions of trauma quickly moved to accounts of the centrality of trauma in both AOD abuse and mental health problems for many women and attendant stories of trauma's neglect in both mental health and AOD service settings. The process evaluation also confirmed that CSRs in this project's target population prefer an approach that incorporates simultaneous attention to their multiple problems. Further, CSRs prefer that multiple services be offered at the same site as long as appropriate measures are taken to assure confidentiality. At the *systems* level, fragmentation between the mental health and AOD service systems is evident in difficulties with cross-referrals, in separate funding streams, in exclusion of people with severe mental health problems from AOD programs and of people with AOD problems from mental health programs, and in incompatible treatment philosophies. Coordination among programs and agencies is therefore necessary to sustain an integrated approach for individual CSRs.

3. Provide a comprehensive range of core services. In addition to the specific absence of trauma services, other necessary supports for women in the target population are often unavailable. Our Phase I process evaluation and systems assessment found especially a paucity of parenting and peer-run services and a scarcity of housing and supported housing programs.

4. Involve CSRs in central roles. One of the key principles of a trauma-informed approach to services is the development of collaborative relationships between CSRs and providers in which power is shared and CSR perspectives are valued. In most service settings for the project population, CSRs have little involvement in planning, implementing, or evaluating services.

5. Are sensitive to issues of gender and culture. A considerable body of literature and clinical experience support the necessity of addressing the unique concerns of women in relationship to mental health, AOD, and trauma difficulties (e.g., Harris, 1994, 1996). In our predominantly African American city and study sample, culturally competent services are a necessity as well (Millet, 1997).

6. Provide additional needed services and integration, including those related to HIV needs. In addition to mental health, AOD, and trauma services, CSRs need a wide range of other supports: housing assistance, help with entitlement and other benefit programs, vocational supports, child care, etc. These fundamental needs often must be addressed in order for women to use other services effectively. We also recognize the additional contributions that abuse histories as well as mental health and drug or alcohol abuse problems make to HIV-risk behavior and to self-care for those women who are HIV-positive (Goodman & Fallot, 1998).

PURPOSE AND GOALS

In response to these needs, the DCTCS developed Integrated Trauma Services Teams (ITSTs) in two human service agencies in D.C., Community Connections and Lutheran Social Services of the National Capital Area. ITSTs are based on the principles of the Trauma Recovery and Empowerment Model (TREM), a fully manualized and clinically tested approach to work with women abuse survivors (Harris, 1998; Fallot & Harris, 2002). These teams provide an integrated, comprehensive package of services aimed at strengthening survivors' trauma recovery skills while simultaneously addressing mental health and AOD problems. Recovery skill development and enhancement on one side are thus coupled with reduction of mental health symptoms and reduction in alcohol and other drug use on the other. Embedded in a trauma-informed network of programs offering a full range of necessary support services, ITSTs are comprised of primary clinicians cross-trained in trauma, AOD, and mental health domains. The teams provide services addressing these domains and the complex interactions among them concurrently and in a closely coordinated way.

In several ways, the ITSTs place trauma recovery skills at the center of service delivery: (1) collaborative and ongoing assessments focus on the eleven skill dimensions comprising the Trauma Recovery and Empowerment Profile (TREP) developed for this project; (2) primary clinicians emphasize recovery skill development in each service contact; (3) each woman in the project participates in a 33-session TREM group with its parallel self-help workbook. Both TREM and the project's other trauma-informed groups (i.e., AOD, parenting, spirituality, HIV support, domestic violence) are explicitly integrative and skills-focused. In addition, project CSRs developed a Women's Support and Empowerment Center offering hospitality, advocacy, peer-led groups, and other activities. Coordinated by CSR leaders with the support of professional staff, this Center provides a welcoming environment for new project participants, mutual support in recovery, and activities planned and led primarily by CSRs.

TARGET POPULATION

We have described the target population for our project in articles based on surveys conducted at Community Connections in the last decade. Goodman et al. (1995) reported the prevalence and types of physical and sexual assault among women at the agency. Fully 87% of the women reported physical abuse in childhood and 87% in adulthood; 65% reported childhood sexual abuse and 76% adult sexual abuse. Severe forms of abuse were by far the most common. Co-occurrence rates indicate the virtual universality of abuse experiences in this urban population of poor women: 92% had been abused physically or sexually, or both, in childhood and 92% had been abused in adulthood. Over their lifetimes, 97% of the women had been sexually or physically abused or both. Second, our surveys (Goodman et al., 1997) found that recent victimization was prevalent in the target population with nearly 30% experiencing abuse in the last month. And recent victimization in turn was related to symptom severity. Even for women with very extensive trauma histories, new experiences of violence exacerbate life difficulties. Finally, we found that histories of abuse increase risk for AOD problems and other HIV-risk behaviors among women in this group (Goodman & Fallot, 1998).

All women served by the ITSTs have a diagnosed mental disorder; it is an eligibility criterion for these publicly funded programs. Twenty to 25% have a schizophrenia spectrum diagnosis and 70% are diagnosed with affective disorders, mostly major depression or bipolar disorders. In the overall population at project sites, approximately 70-75% of consumers have a substance use disorder. Of those individuals with a substance use disorder, almost 90% meet the criteria for an alcohol abuse disorder. Over 50% have abused cocaine (usually crack) and virtually all of these individuals also have abused alcohol. Fewer than 5% of the women consumers at the ITST programs have primary caretaking responsibilities for their children. While nearly 60% of the women have had children, almost 70% of the children are over 18 years of age.

Over 85% of the women are African American with 10-15% European American; there are few Latina and Asian women receiving services at these agencies. Our surveys indicate no significant ethnic differences between African American and European American women in rates of physical or sexual abuse. This is consistent with other published studies assessing multiple ethnic groups (Roosa et al., 1999; Arroyo et al., 1997; Dansky et al., 1996). Research by Boyd et al. (1997) focused on African American women using crack cocaine and found rates of sexual trauma similar to the overall patterns described above. Similarly, our data describing ITST consumers indicate no significant ethnic/cultural variations in the rates of specific mental health or substance use disorders.

DEVELOPMENT OF THE INTERVENTION

Pre-study surveys and clinical experience. As described above, our surveys found very high, almost universal, rates of trauma among women with substance use and mental disorders. In addition, we confirmed that violent victimization increases the risk for a host of other problems in both alcohol and other drug abuse and mental health domains, including HIV-risk behavior. Clinical work and literature reviews demonstrated the complex roles violence plays for women survivors in relationship to AOD and mental health problems. For example, for many women alcohol and other substances help to manage trauma-related emotional states, soothing in response to distress or anxiety and stimulating in response to depression or numbness. Substance use, however, also is connected to increased risk of revictimization, especially by involvement in unsafe networks and relationships. Further, it became clear that trauma histories complicate engagement and continuation in services; women felt unwelcome and often left services that were not sensitive to the breadth and depth of trauma's impact on their lives. These formal and informal findings coincided with the development not only of a trauma-specific group intervention (TREM) but to a focus on ensuring a trauma-informed setting for project participants.

The development of the TREM group intervention. For several years prior to the initiation of the DCTCS, clinicians at Community Connections led by Maxine Harris, the agency's Clinical Director, developed and refined the 33-session group intervention. The planning group of nearly 20 women clinicians selected topics for each session; set specific session goals; and developed discussion questions and exercises designed to meet those goals. In collaboration with consumer-survivors who participated in the initial groups and provided specific feedback about the session's appropriateness and helpfulness, the planners then included, discarded, and refined sessions until the final set of 33 sessions was selected and described in detail. The manualized version of TREM, with session-by-session guidelines for group leaders, was published in 1998 (Harris, 1998).

Pilot studies of the TREM groups built on this early experience and focused on several questions: the feasibility of the group, including the question of fidelity measurement; its attractiveness to consumer-survivors; and its potential risks and benefits. At Community Connections, we conducted qualitative individual and group discussions with TREM leaders, participants, and other clinicians over several years to address these questions and gathered preliminary quantitative data regarding possible benefits. In addition, as TREM was implemented in other settings, we conducted informal evaluations reflecting the priorities of these programs and the group participants. In terms of *feasibility* in these various sites, administrators consistently recognized the need for trauma recovery services and expressed support for including TREM in their programs. Many clinicians voiced strong interest in leading TREM groups and group leaders participated in a three-day training that included a session-by-session explanation of the intervention as well as demonstrations and practice of leader skills. They reported that this training, coupled with ongoing supervision or consultation, provided them with the necessary skills to lead groups effectively. Finally, we developed a TREM Fidelity Scale to assess the consistency and quality of the group's implementation. This instrument measures key elements of the treatment context (e.g., clinician support for member participation, appropriateness of screening and referral) and samples leader behavior (e.g., activity level, educational and problem-solving foci, goal accomplishment, and leadership style). Raters readily came to consensus ratings of observed and audiotaped group sessions.

The *attractiveness* of TREM was confirmed in high rates of enrollment; very few women (less than 10% in most settings) approached to participate in the groups declined to do so after hearing a description of its content and style. And most of the women who declined cited, not the trauma-focused content, but the length of the group as a potential difficulty for them. Retention and completion rates for the group were also high. In our surveys, across a variety of sites, approximately 70% of women completed more than 75% of the TREM sessions. These findings contrasted markedly with a significant concern of some administrators and clinicians that trauma-focused interventions would lead to consumer distress and increased drop-out.

Several of the informal evaluations addressed *consumer satisfaction* with the groups directly. Over 95% of the participants reported that the group was helpful to them. When asked about specifics, group members in one agency reported that they felt support from other group members (95%), experienced "more control over" their lives (95%), were more able to assert themselves (85%), and were involved in safer relationships (79%).

Finally, in terms of *potential risks and benefits*, we found very few adverse responses to TREM groups in these pilot projects. Women who discontinued usually said that they did not like group approaches in general; they did not report that the trauma content as a significant factor. Although any discussion of trauma is potentially distressing for group members, group members reported that the present-day, empowerment, and coping skill emphases of TREM groups minimize this possibility. On the other hand, potential benefits included reported decreases in alcohol and other drug abuse, mental health symptoms, and utilization of intensive services like emergency rooms and inpatient hospitalizations. There were corresponding increases in clinician ratings of overall functioning, safety, and recovery skill development (Fallot & Harris, 2001).

The development of a trauma-informed service context. Being trauma-informed involves fundamental shifts in both thinking and practice, a paradigm change from traditional understandings of trauma, the consumer-survivor, services, and services relationship (Harris & Fallot, 2001). For the DCTCS, this meant embedding the TREM group intervention in a fully trauma-informed context, the Integrated Trauma Services Teams. A setting that is trauma-informed incorporates several basic principles about trauma. First, profound and repeated abuse is seen as a life-altering event that affects a woman's development and functioning across the life-span and has an impact on a wide range of areas of functioning. Second, current symptoms are viewed as attempts to understand, cope with, or defend against the impact of trauma and as such may represent a woman's strength and creative coping capacities. Finally, problems and solutions are best approached from an integrated, holistic, whole person perspective and require the full collaboration of consumers in the development of goals that are empowerment and growth oriented.

Five guiding principles are especially central to trauma-informed settings: consumer emotional and physical safety; consumer choice and control; clarity of consumer and staff tasks and boundaries; collaboration and power-sharing between consumers and staff; and consumer empowerment and skill-building (Fallot & Harris, 2002a). The DCTCS agencies, especially the immediate ITST context, placed emphasis on these principles in all aspects of service delivery. Standard guidelines for resource coordination and advocacy were adapted to prioritize the fundamental shifts in both clinical understanding and daily practice reflected in the trauma-informed paradigm.

The importance of gender-specificity. Mental health, AOD, and trauma programming have become increasingly aware of the unique needs of women (Amaro & Hardy-Fanta, 1995; Harris, 1997; Levin et al., 1998; Underhill & Finnegan, 1996). Recurring recommendations in this literature include the importance of women's choice and control; emphasizing women's strengths; offering a safe and supportive environment; providing women-only services; being non-confrontational in style; focusing on women's relationships in all services; teaching specific life skills and coping strategies; and fostering caring relationships with staff and other consumers. Two themes were especially important for the development of the DCTCS. The first is a priority on *empowerment* and a *strengths-based* orientation in women's services. Feminist principles emphasizing women's specific coping skills and capacities for adaptation have guided service development in both AOD and trauma arenas (Abbott, 1994; Harris, 1998). The reframing of many "symptoms" as having originated in understandable attempts to cope with trauma (e.g., dissociation as a valuable survival technique) is a key part of the TREM approach, for example.

The second theme for women's programming addresses the significance and power of understanding women's development, strengths, and coping skills in the context of *relationships*. Services for women need to take seriously the role of key relationships in both the development and maintenance of problems (such as the abuse of alcohol and other substances) and in the process of recovery (e.g., Amaro & Hardy-Fanta, 1995). Especially in a sociocultural context that often devalues women and sees relational priorities as weakness, one important implication of this recognition is the value of offering women same-sex services (e.g., Abel et al., 1996). Groups like TREM that build on group cohesiveness and shared experiences of women members can demonstrate the power of supportive relationships in recovery (Harris, 1998).

The importance of cultural competence. While overall trauma rates may not differ among racial and cultural subgroups of women, the *meaning* of abuse and the unique consequences are essential considerations in the development of effective services. For African American women with complex histories of trauma, poverty, and frequent homelessness in addition to AOD and mental health problems, this array of concerns must be placed against a history of race-based oppression, discrimination, and marginalization. The result is often not only a sense of disempowerment but of culturally sanctioned silence. Millet (1997) has detailed some of the unique concerns facing African American women trauma survivors. For example, sensitivity to the frequent reluctance of African American women to discuss family violence is essential, given the dilemma they often experience of responsibility for keeping families together even if this unity comes at the expense of denying or minimizing family-based abuse (Greene, 1994).

We incorporated other key elements of these culturally focused findings in both the ITSTs and the TREM groups. Both, for example, value empowerment in a way reflective of cultural issues. The TREM group approach was developed in a collaborative way, based heavily on the responses of predominantly African American group members. The group members themselves reported what was helpful and unhelpful about the approach and significantly contributed to its final shape and content. Culture-specific elements include the use of language that fits the participants; words and phrases used by group members to describe their experiences were incorporated in the manual and culturally appropriate materials are used in group exercises. In addition, the groups themselves often become alternative support resources for many members and this extra-group contact is reinforced. In order to give more attention to the place of religion and spirituality in African American culture, project staff members from the two agencies collaborated in developing a manualized, 11-session group addressing the role of spirituality in recovery from trauma.

ROLE OF CONSUMER/SURVIVOR/RECOVERING PERSONS

CSRs played key roles in three distinct aspects of the development and implementation of the DCTCS. First, as noted above, consumer-survivors participated actively in the development of the core TREM intervention. They provided direct feedback to group leaders about the content, structure, and process of the preliminary versions of the group. This feedback in turn was incorporated in subsequent versions of TREM and these were then evaluated by both group members and leaders until a final version of TREM was published. Second, in Phase I of the project, CSRs formed an advisory group called the "Empowered Survivors Council." This group of 15-20 CSRs collectively and individually played a central part in the planning and implementation of our Phase II intervention and evaluation research. As a group, the Empowered Survivors Council made recommendations about the role of CSRs on the project; planned peer support activities; collaborated on recruiting and the informed consent process; and worked to welcome new participants into the project. Individually, members joined other working committees focused on trauma screening, training and education, evaluation, and systems assessment. CSRs became paid members of the project staff as Consumer Coordinator, as Consumer Advocate/Researcher, and as Peer Support Specialists. In terms of educational activities, CSRs have been active throughout the project in using the *Women Speak Out* video developed by Community Connections to highlight the prevalence and impact of trauma in women's lives and to discuss paths to empowerment and recovery. CSRs drew on this video in offering training for providers in trauma-related issues and in presenting their experiences to other consumers who might be interested in the project. Finally, in Phase II, CSRs worked to develop a peer-run drop-in center for women called the Women's Support and Empowerment Center. This space serves not only welcoming and peer support functions but offers a range of individual and group activities initiated by CSR women (see the section on services below).

DESCRIPTION OF THE INTERVENTIONS

Structurally, each ITST consists of four to six clinicians and a clinical supervisor. Each CSR, upon entry into the program, begins working with her primary clinician on an Integrated Assessment, a Personal Recovery Plan, and the integration and coordination of all services. The task of the primary clinician is to assist each CSR to meet her Recovery Plan goals by drawing on the CSR's personal strengths; on a comprehensive array of professional and consumer-led services; and on other community resources. Clinicians on the team all become acquainted with each CSR in order to provide team backup and additional support.

The assessment follows standard guidelines for assessing mental and physical health, AOD, residential, vocational, financial and relational concerns. Together, the consumer and clinician identify goals and potential barriers as they work toward making progress in each of these areas. The assessment does not stop with the standard target domains, however. For each consumer, a team member completes a Trauma Recovery and Empowerment Profile (TREP) as part of the initial assessment process. We have identified eleven areas of skill development that are essential to recovery from the impact of prolonged trauma among people with severe mental disorders and AOD abuse:

- *Self-awareness*–the ability to recognize bodily and motivational states and to articulate that awareness to others in a clear manner;
- *Self-protection*–the ability to recognize, avoid, and/or manage potentially harmful situations and to establish safe and manageable interpersonal boundaries;
- *Self-soothing*–the ability to mange and diminish feelings of distress, pain, and hurt;
- *Emotional modulation*–strategies to control the intensity and expression of affective states;
- *Relational mutuality*–the capacity to engage in a reciprocal meeting of interpersonal needs;
- *Accurate labeling of self and others*–the capacity to use accurate words to label one's own behavior and the behavior of others;
- *Sense of agency and initiative-taking*–the ability to see oneself as the primary source of action and initiative in one's life;
- *Consistent problem solving*–the ability to combine cognitive, affective and social skills in resolving personal and interpersonal situations;
- *Reliable parenting*–the ability to respond to the needs of dependent children and grandchildren in a reliable and consistent way;
- *Possessing a sense of purpose and meaning*–the ability to actively seek and meet one's needs in an appropriate manner and to view one's actions in a larger context of meaning;
- *Judgment and decision making*–the ability to form reliable judgments based on thoughts, feelings, and perceptions and to use those judgments to make beneficial decisions.

The Trauma Recovery and Empowerment Profile (TREP) includes five-point behaviorally anchored rating scales for each of the eleven recovery skill dimensions. Team members work with consumers not only to complete the initial profile but also to prioritize skill areas for ongoing recovery work. No more than four skill domains are designated as primary areas of emphasis. ITST members use a manual of skill development exercises to assist consumers with skill-building in their chosen priority areas. Clinicians collaborate with CSRs to provide education about trauma, mental health, and AOD problems; to appropriately reframe current symptoms as trauma-related coping attempts; to facilitate basic skill development in self-protection, self-regulation, boundary maintenance, and communications and relationship development.

For each woman, the TREP and standard assessments help to identify areas of individualized concern. Consumers and clinicians design a plan together targeted at accomplishing the goals identified by the dual assessments. Regardless of the consumer-specific interventions that might be devised, however, each consumer is exposed to the TREM intervention which forms the core of the DCTCS project.

The TREM intervention is a 33-session group designed to meet weekly for 75 minutes each session. Up to twelve women and two to three co-facilitators progress through the curriculum using a combination of active discussion and experiential exercises to accomplish the goals of each session. The intervention is divided into three separate components: an empowerment section that helps women to acquire or reinforce the skills, such as limit-setting and self-soothing, necessary for active recovery; a trauma recovery module designed to address the specific sequelae of sexual and physical abuse; and a skills enhancement section targeted at helping women develop practical skills in communication, problem solving and emotional modulation. The following are key elements of the TREM group approach:

- Basic education about physical and sexual abuse and how current behaviors are linked to past abuses;
- A reframing of current symptoms as attempts to cope with unbearable trauma;
- An appreciation for the problem-solving attempts locked and hidden in certain repetitive behaviors;
- Education focusing on basic skills in self-regulation, boundary maintenance, and communication;
- Basic education about female sexuality, correcting misperceptions and misconceptions;

- Creation of a healing community by providing recovery services within a group;
- Rediscovery of and reconnection to lost memories, feelings, and perceptions;
- An opportunity for women to experience a sense of competence and resolution as they face the demons from the past; and
- An opportunity for women to trust their own perceptions about reality and to receive validation from others for those correct perceptions.

TREM groups draw on a range of techniques shown to be effective in facilitating trauma recovery; cognitive restructuring, skills training, psychoeducation, and peer support are primary intervention methods (Fallot & Harris, 2002b). For women who are unable to complete the TREM intervention in the prescribed group format a self-help version was developed and made available, allowing women to work on the topics alone or with a clinician or peer companion. All participants in the study were given an S-TREM book, *Healing the Trauma of Abuse,* (Copeland & Harris, 2000) and even women who attended the groups regularly often chose to reinforce the group learning by reviewing the topics on their own.

In addition to the TREM groups, women were offered a variety of other groups that complemented and built on the skills developed in the TREM groups. These offerings, all of which were voluntary, included the following:

1. *Spirituality in Trauma Recovery.* This group addresses spiritual and religious resources for empowerment and recovery from physical and sexual abuse. After reviewing group members' spiritual histories and the possible relations between religion/spirituality and trauma, sessions focus on such topics as spiritual models and activities, spiritually nourishing communities, and spiritual responses to painful events and relationships.

2. *Domestic Violence.* The group focuses specifically on understanding the cycle of violence within a relationship and developing ways to stop the cycle. Specific topics include anger, assertiveness, power and control, and communication skills.

3. *AOD Treatment for Trauma Survivors.* This group focuses on explicit connections for women between trauma sequelae and symptoms and patterns in the use and abuse of alcohol and other drugs. The role of substances as a way to manage intense affect, flashbacks, etc., is discussed. Women also see the links between use patterns and further vic-

timization. Finally, women learn that by recognizing trauma-related symptoms, they can devise alternative strategies for managing those symptoms that do not include the use of substances.

4. *Relapse Prevention.* The group focuses on the development of cognitive and behavioral skills for managing relapse. Specific techniques are employed to manage feelings, recognize triggers, control destructive thinking, and ultimately control behavior.

5. *Trauma Issues and HIV Infection.* For women who are HIV infected, this group attempts to integrate what a woman has learned about her trauma history with strategies for handling her diagnosis of HIV sero-positivity. Women explore how responses to trauma such as self-blame and secrecy might resurface with an HIV diagnosis. Women are given strategies for managing their medical condition and for not letting trauma responses interfere with seeking good medical care.

6. *Parenting.* Three distinct parenting groups are offered. One, for women who are currently parenting their children, focuses on skill development. A second emphasizes the potential impediments to parenting that may arise as a result of having a personal history of abuse and violent victimization and the third is intended for women who are mothers but are not currently parenting and who are dealing with issues of loss and separation.

In addition to the ITSTs and the various group interventions, all consumers have access to psychiatric care and appropriate medications for symptom management. In the event of a psychiatric crisis, consumers can make use of the 24-hour crisis line and speak to a clinician who has been trained to understand trauma symptoms. In the event of a hospitalization, consumers have the choice of several inpatient facilities in the Washington, D.C., area, including the Washington Hospital Center. This unit offers trauma survivors a set of four psycho-educational groups developed in collaboration with the DCTCS; topics include safety planning, trauma and AOD or mental health problems, self-soothing and emotional modulation, and referral for appropriate services.

Finally, the DCTCS offers a range of services that were developed and sponsored by the CSRs in the project. Consumer-run activities are housed in the Women's Support and Empowerment Center, the focal point of CSR involvement. For several hours each day, the Center is open for women to come and meet with others for conversation, support or respite. Peer representatives who staff the Center offer child care, sponsor luncheons for mutual support and networking, and distribute a resource booklet describing available support services and leisure activities. Center staff also offer a selection of wellness activities to project participants. Specific content depends on participant interest and may include the following: swimming, walking, nutrition, cooking, stretching/body movement, massage, gospel singing, gardening, and a variety of crafts activities.

Throughout the project, consumers convened an Empowered Survivors Council that met regularly to discuss the status of the project and to offer suggestions about needed services. Through the Council, peers were available to talk with women referred to the project. Peer representatives helped clarify and describe the services offered and the project goals from a CSR perspective, helping to ensure that consent is fully informed, to debrief after interviews, and to enhance the engagement process.

As a result of consumer input, groups were added at the Women's Support and Empowerment Center on topics such as anger management, self-soothing and self-control, and open discussion. Generally these groups, which were consumer led, were attended by four to six women at a time who used a curriculum to guide their discussions, but who also provided one another with an open and supportive context in which to discuss their concerns and their progress.

LESSONS LEARNED

Conversations with consumers and clinicians taught us that several areas of concern need to be addressed in future projects designed to help women recover from the long-term effects of physical and sexual abuse.

The importance of a trauma-informed context. The core clinical intervention in the DCTCS was the Trauma Recovery and Empowerment Model group. This group was developed to be responsive to the needs of women with multiple vulnerabilities and often unrecognized strengths. It is clear, though, that the impact of this group experience for women with such extensive trauma histories, mental health problems, and substance use difficulties could only be maximized in a trauma-informed context. The primary clinicians in the ITSTs maintained a steady emphasis on trauma throughout service delivery: from recovery planning using the TREP to corresponding skills development in each clinical contact to consistent attention to the key attributes of a trauma-informed setting. These markers of trauma-informed programs–ensuring emotional and physical safety, maximizing consumer choice and control, enhancing clarity of tasks and boundaries, prioritizing collaboration and sharing of power, and facilitating empowerment and skill-building–not only characterized the activities of the ITSTs but of the larger agency service settings. Without such a context, the impact of the TREM groups for women in this target population would likely be significantly compromised.

Safe housing. Without access to permanent, affordable and safe housing, many women expressed the fear that they would be forced to return to abusive partners or family members, despite having learned skills for keeping themselves safe. Especially in large urban areas, where real estate prices are high, many poor women feel permanently marginalized in the housing market. Dreams of re-unification with children seem elusive when women cannot gain access to acceptable housing. As the DCTCS project moved into its third year, Community Connections applied for and was awarded status as a housing authority through the Department of Housing and Urban Development. This allowed several of the women in the project to complete successful applications for Section 8 housing vouchers. As women moved into safe neighborhoods, they felt freer to begin using many of the skills they had acquired as a result of TREM participation.

Booster groups. Many women who successfully completed TREM groups expressed a desire to either repeat the group in its entirety or to participate in periodic booster sessions. Women confided that even when they attended every group, they often missed important content because they were overwhelmed by feelings or intrusive thoughts during the group. Women also expressed a need to remain part of a community of survivors who were also engaged in active recovery work. Some women felt that as they progressed, both mentally and physically, they were able to appreciate the content of the TREM groups more fully and at a deeper level. These women believed that repeating the group would almost be like taking it for the first time because they now saw themselves and others with such different eyes. If recovery is to be ongoing, it seems reasonable that some ongoing access to TREM groups be available to those who want to participate.

Advanced relationship work. The greatest risk for relapse (either mental health or drug related) lies in the complicated world of interpersonal relationships. At the beginning of the trauma project, most women struggled with the maintenance of secure emotional and physical boundaries. As they learned new skills for how to stay safe, many opted for at least a temporary hiatus from the world of relationships, choosing to avoid past abusers and to stay aloof from new relationships. Initially this avoidance strategy worked well to keep women safe while they focused on trauma recovery issues and worked to develop new coping skills. Over time, however, as women saw their lives achieving a level of stability and calm never before experienced, many began to articulate feelings of profound and pervasive loneliness. Regrettably, some felt that the only salve for the emptiness they felt was to return to past relationships, often with a past abuser. Some, however, voiced a desire for more intensive recovery work, focusing specifically on the pitfalls and perils of re-establishing all-important interpersonal connectedness without encountering further abuse. These women have been meeting with a group of clinicians to design an advanced recovery curriculum that will address their current needs for safe relationships.

REFERENCES

Abbott, A. A. (1994). A feminist approach to substance abuse treatment and service delivery. *Social Work Health Care, 19*(304), 67-83.

Abel, K., Buszewicz, M., Davison, S., Johnson, S., & Staples, E. (Eds.). (1996). *Planning Community Mental Health Services for Women: A Multiprofessional Handbook*. London: Routledge.

Amaro, H., & Hardy-Fanta, C. (1995). Gender relations in addiction and recovery. *Journal of Psychoactive Drugs, 27*(4), 325-327.

Arroyo, J. A., Simpson, T. L., & Aragon, A. S. (1997). Childhood sexual abuse among Hispanic and non-Hispanic White college women. *Hispanic Journal of Behavioral Sciences, 19*(1), 57-68.

Boyd, C., Henderson, D., Ross-Durow, P., & Aspen, J. (1997). Sexual trauma and depression in African-American women who smoke crack cocaine. *Substance Abuse, 18*(3), 133-141.

Copeland, M. E., & Harris, M. (2000). *Healing the Trauma of Abuse: A Women's Workbook*. Oakland, CA: New Harbinger Publications, Inc.

Dansky, B. S., Brady, K. T., Saladin, M. E., Killeen, T., Becker, S., & Roitzsch, J. (1996). Victimization and PTSD in individuals with substance use disorders: Gender and racial differences. *American Journal of Drug and Alcohol Abuse, 22*(1), 75-93.

Fallot, R. D. (1997). Spirituality in trauma recovery. In Harris, M. (Ed.) *Sexual Abuse in the Lives of Women Diagnosed with Serious Mental Illness* (pp. 337-355). Netherlands: Harwood Academic Publishers.

Fallot, R. D., & Harris, M. (2002a). *Trauma-Informed Services: A Self-Assessment and Planning Protocol*. Community Connections.

Fallot, R. D., & Harris, M. (2002b). The Trauma Recovery and Empowerment Model (TREM): Conceptual and practical issues in a group intervention for women. *Community Mental Health Journal, 38*(6), 475-485.

Goodman, L. A., Dutton, M. A., & Harris, M. (1995). Physical and sexual assault prevalence among episodically homeless women with serious mental illness. *American Journal of Orthopsychiatry, 65*(4), 468-478.

Goodman, L. A., & Fallot, R. D. (1998). HIV risk-behavior in poor urban women with serious mental disorders: Association with childhood physical and sexual abuse. *American Journal of Orthopsychiatry, 68*, 73-83.

Greene, B. (1994). *African American Women, Women of Color: Integrating Ethnic and Gender Identities in Psychotherapy.* New York: Guilford Press.

Harris, M. (1994). Modifications in service delivery and clinical treatment for women diagnosed with severe mental illness who are also the survivors of sexual abuse trauma. *Journal of Mental Health Administration, 21,* 397-406.

Harris, M. (1996). Treating sexual abuse trauma with dually diagnosed women. *Community Mental Health Journal, 32*(4).

Harris, M. (Ed.). (1997). *Sexual Abuse in the Lives of Women Diagnosed with Serious Mental Illness.* Netherlands: Harwood Academic Publishers.

Harris, M. (1998). *Trauma Recovery and Empowerment: A Clinician's Guide for Working with Women in Groups.* New York, NY: The Free Press.

Harris, M. (2001). *A Menu of Strategies for Improving a Woman's Trauma Recovery and Empowerment Profile.* Community Connections.

Harris, M., & Fallot, R. D. (Eds.). (2001). *Using Trauma Theory to Design Service Systems. New Directions for Mental Health Services.* San Francisco: Jossey-Bass.

Levin, B. L., Blanch, A. K., & Jennings, A. (Eds.). (1998). *Women's Mental Health Services: A Public Health Perspective.* Thousand Oaks, CA: Sage.

Lincoln, C. E., & Mamiya, L. H. (1990). *The Black Church in the African American Experience.* New York: Duke University Press.

Millet, B. L. (1997). Sexual trauma and African American women. In Harris, M. *Sexual Abuse in the Lives of Women Diagnosed with Serious Mental Illness* (pp. 321-336). Netherlands: Harwood Academic Publisher.

Roosa, M. W., Reinholtz, C., & Angelini, P. J. (1999). The relation of child sexual abuse and depression in young women: comparisons across four ethnic groups. *Journal of Abnormal and Child Psychology, 27*(1), 65-.

Underhill, B. L., & Finnegan, D. G. (Eds.). (1996). *Chemical Dependency: Women at Risk.* Binghamton, NY: Harrington Park Press.

Index

Adaptive strategies, 6
Advocacy, 55,73-74
Agency, sense of, 192
Agency-level integration, 68-69
Alcoholics Anonymous, 90
Allies Program, 161-180
   background and principles, 162
   client engagement, 177
   conclusions, 178
   cross-discipline integration, 175
   CSRs in, 170-171,175-176
   environmental context, 163
   goals, 164
   implementation: individual level,
      172-175
   implementation: systems level,
      171-172
   intervention: individual-level,
      166-170
   intervention: systems-level,
      165-166
   intervention development, 165-170
   lessons learned, 175-178
   parenting curriculum, 169-170
   problem statement, 162-163
   resource limitations, 178
   service coordination, 168-169
   service provider training and
      support, 176-177
   target population, 164
   trauma-specific services, 166-168
Arapahoe House Directions for
      Families Program (Denver),
      141-160
   background and principles, 142
   child care issues, 153
   children's services, 154,157

   community services, 158
   CSRs in, 155-156
   employment/vocational services,
      152-153
   history, 144-145
   housing issues, 152-153
   intervention services, 149-156
   lessons learned, 156-159
   mental health services, 150
   need for integration, 143-144
   parenting services, 154
   phases of intervention, 148-149
   philosophy, 145-148
   POWER program, 148-149,156,
      158-159
   problem statement, 142-143
   skills and recovery development I,
      149-155
   target population, 145,146
   transitional issues, 157-158
   trauma-specific services, 150-151
Assessment, 106-107,132-133
ATRIUM Model, 29
Attendance issues, 55

Basic life skills, 152
Bavolek's Nurturing Program. *See*
      Nurturing Program
Booster groups, 197
Boston Consortium of Services, 12-13,
      95-119
   background and principles, 96-97
   client participation and retention,
      113
   client participation tracking, 112
   conclusion, 114-115

CSRs in, 104,110
cultural/linguistic adaptation,
    113-114
data collection, 102
developmental research, 102-103
evaluation issues, 112
expert consultants, 111-112
implementation challenges,
    109-114
intervention development, 101-108
interventions: individual level,
    106-108
interventions: system level,
    104-106
intervention sites, 108-109
leadership issues, 109-110
literature review, 97-98
outpatient treatment programs,
    108-109
race/ethnic differences, 99-101
residential treatment, 108
staff training, 111
sustained communication
    mechanisns, 110
target population, 98-101
workgroup structures, 111
Brief Symptoms Inventory (Derogatis),
    49

California, San Joaquin County Allies
    Program, 161-180. *See also*
    Allies Program
CalWORKS. *See* PROTOTYPES
    centers
Cambridge, Masssachusetts study, 12,
    19-39. *See also* Franklin
    County Women's Research
    Project
Case management, 168-169,173-174
Challenges and rewards, of CSR
    training, 35-36
Child care issues, 131,137,153
Children's services, 157

Clark, Colleen, xiv
Client participation tracking, 112
Cognitive-behavioral approach,
    146-147
Colorado study, 141-160. *See also*
    Arapahoe House Directions
    for Families Program
Communication, sustained, 110
Community Connections, 181-199
Community Consensus Building
    Collaborative, 66
Community development, 31-32
Community Initiatives Grants, 32
Community services, 158
Co-morbidity Resource Card, 106
Co-morbidity screening, 106
Consumer Advisory Board, Triad
    Women's Project, 55-56
Consumer Advisory Committees, 135
Consumer integration, 71-72. *See also*
    CSRs
Consumer/survivor/recovering women.
    See CSRs
Continuity of care, 54,157-158
Countertransference, 138
County programs, San Joaquin County
    Allies Program, 161-180. *See
    also* Allies Program
Cross-training, 67-68,105-106,175
CSRs, 110
    Allies Program, 170-171,175-176
    Arapahoe House Directions for
        Families Program, 155-156
    challenges and rewards, 35-36
    Franklin County (MA) Women's
        Research Project, 32-33
    Integrated Trauma Services Teams,
        191
    Portal Project, 134-135
    PROTOTYPES centers, 89-92
Cultural competence, 131,190. *See
    also* Ethnicity and culture
Cultural/linguistic adaptation, 113-114
Cultural sensitivity, 52

Decision making, 192
Demographics. *See* Target population
Denver study, 13,141-160. *See also*
    Arapahoe House Directions
    for Families Program
Derogatis Brief Symptom Inventory, 49
Disempowerment, 25-26
Distress Tolerance, 53
District of Columbia Trauma
    Collaboration Study,
    181-199. *See also* Integrated
    Trauma Services Teams
Domestic violence, 194
Double Trouble twelve-step program,
    66
Drop-In Centers, 28-29
Drugs of choice, 73,101

Economic Success in Recovery, 107
Emotional modulation, 192
Emotional Regulation, 53
Employment and vocational services,
    152-153
Empowerment, 189
Entre Familia residential program, 108
Ethnicity and culture, 45-46,52,97-98,
    98-101,131-132,190
ETR Associates, 161-180
Evaluation issues, 112
Expert consultants, 111-112

Families, Allies Program, 174-175
Family Nurturing Program, 107-108
Family/social support, 153-154
Federal response, 3-4
Flexibility, 52
Florida Center for Addictions and Dual
    Disorders, 41-61
Franklin County (MA) Women's
    Research Project, 19-39
    ATRIUM Model, 29
    background and principles, 10-21
    clinical/individual services, 30
    community development, 31-32
    conclusion, 36
    CSR program, 32-33
    Drop-In Center, 28-29
    heuristic model, 26-28
    individual responses, 23
    intervention description, 25-32
    lessons learned, 33-36
    organizational/program integration,
        30-31
    overview, 21-23
    Peer Resource Advocates, 29-30
    policy and practice committees, 31
    purpose and goals, 25
    rural services provision, 22
    service model, 28-32
    systems and services integration,
        21-22
    target population, 23-24
    theoretical underpinnings, 25-28

Gender-specific services, 52,189-190
Goals, of entire study, 9-10
Griffin House residential center, 108

Haitian women, ethnic and cultural
    studies, 45-46
Handbook for Triad Mothers (Kuehnle
    & Becker), 57
Healing the Trauma of Abuse
    (Copeland & Harris), 194
Healthy-lifestyle modeling, 156-157
Helping Women Recover (Covington),
    87-88
Herman's stages of recovery, 25-26
Herman's Trauma and Recovery
    Model, 167
Hispanic women, in Triad Women's
    Project, 45-46
Housing issues, 152-153,197
Human potential movement, 25
Hunter College School of Social Work,
    121-139

Implementation challenges, 109-114
Individual recovery, 149-152
Initiative-taking, 192
Institute for Health and Recovery
　　　(Cambridge, MA), 64. *See
　　　also* WELL project
Integrated Trauma Services Teams,
　　　181-199. *See also* TREM
　　　Model
　　background and principles, 182
　　CSRs in, 191
　　intervention description, 191-196
　　intervention development, 186-190
　　lessons learned, 196-198
　　problem statement, 182-184
　　purpose and goals, 184-185
　　target population, 185-186
Integration, 35
　　agency-level, 68-69
　　barriers to, 91
　　clinical level, 30
　　community-level, 69-70
　　consumer, 71-72
　　cross-training curriculum, 67-68
　　lack of, 66,102-103
　　need for, 183-184
　　services, 30-31
　　state-level, 70-71
Interagency agreements, 105
Interagency service planning, WELL
　　　Project, 74
Internships, 32
Interpersonal Effectiveness and Skills,
　　　53

Jane Doe, Inc., 70
Joint planning, 104-105
Journey Beyond Abuse (Fisher &
　　　McGrane), 151
Judgment, 192

(University of) Kansas, 169

Labeling, of self and others, 192
Leadership issues, 109-110
Lifestyle modeling, 156-157
Local resource mobilization, 34

Maslow's hierarchy of needs, 25
Media relations, 32
Mindfulness, 52-53
Mom's Project outpatient program,
　　　108-109
Multi-Disciplinary Team Case
　　　Conferences, 129

New England Research Institutes,
　　　95-119
Nurturing Program (Bavolek), 76,154,
　　　169-170

Overview of text, 11-13

Palladia, Inc. *See* Portal Project
Paradigm development, 34
Parenting, 75-76,154,169-170,192,195
Peer Councils, 135
Peer-led mutual help groups, 76-77
Peer-led services, 35
Peer Resource Advocates, 29-30
Peer Support groups, 49-50
Phase I activities, 10-11
Phase I goals and objectives, 9
Phase II goals and objectives, 9-10
Policy Action Committees, 129
Portal Project, 121-139
　　administrative/system observations,
　　　137-139
　　background and principles, 122-124
　　clinical assessment, 132-133
　　clinical observations, 136-137
　　CSRs in, 134-135
　　developmental research, 127-128
　　ethnicity and culture, 131-132

intervention descriptions, 130-134
intervention development, 127-129
lessons learned, 136-139
philosophies and principles,
129-130
problem statement, 124-126
purpose and goals, 127
residential treatment, 133-134
system level intervention, 129
target population, 126-127
Therapeutic Community approach,
130-131
Posttraumatic stress disorder (PTSD),
44-45,89-90,133,167
POWER program, 148-149,156,
157-158,158-159
Prevalence, 5
Primary Treatment Network, 172
Problem solving, 192
Project Return Foundation, 121-139
PROTOTYPES centers, 81-95
background and principles, 82-83
CSR integration, 89-92
lessons learned, 92-93
residential treatment model, 87,
88-89
service integration, 86-89
systems integration, 83-86
Purpose, sense of, 192

Race. *See* Ethnicity and culture
Rapp's strength-based case
management, 169
Readiness, 51-52
Recovering Families, Allies Program,
174-175
Recovery, stages of, 26
Relapse prevention, 195
Relational mutuality, 192
Relational Theory, 25,26
Relationship context, 189-190
Relationships, advanced work in,
197-198
Residential treatment

Boston Consortium of Services, 108
Portal Project, 133-134
PROTOTYPES model, 87,88-89
Resource coordination, 55
WELL Project, 73-74
Resource Coordination Councils, 74
Resource sharing, 105
Rural programs, 41-61. *See also* Triad
Women's Project
Rutgers–Newark, 19-39, xiv

Safe housing, 197
SAMHSA, 7-8, xiv-xv
goals and objectives, 11
San Joaquin County Allies Program,
161-180. *See also* Allies
Program
Seeking Safety, 134,136-137,167,
172-174
Seeking Safety (Najavits), 87-88
Self-awareness, 192
Self-protection, 192
Self-soothing, 192
Sense of agency, 192
Sense of purpose, 192
Service delivery issues, 72-77
Service integration. *See* Integration
Service system issues, 2-4. *See also*
Integration
Skills-building groups, 107-108
*Skills Training Manual for Treating
Borderline Personality
Disorder* (Linehan), 48
Social/family support, 153-154
Solution-Focused therapy, 147
(University of) South Florida, 41-61,
xiv
Spirituality, 194
*Staff Handbook for Addressing Parent
Needs* (Kuehnle & Becker),
57
Staff training, 111
Staff turnover, 176-177
Stages of Change model, 145-146

Stanley Street Project and Resources, 65. *See also* WELL Project

State-level integration, 70-71

Stone Center's Relational Theory. *See* Relational Theory

Strength-based approach, 52

Strengths-based approach, 189

Strengths-based case management, 169

Substance abuse, drug of choice, 71

Substance Abuse and Mental Health Services Administration. *See* SAMHSA

Substance Abuse Treatment and Prevention-Addiction Services, 109

Systematic Training for Effective Parenting (STEP) programs, 57

Systems change, levels of, 84

Target population
Allies Program, 164
Arapahoe House Directions for Families Program, 145,146
Boston Consortium of Services, 98-101
of entire study, 9
Franklin County (MA) Women's Research Project, 23-24
Portal Project, 126-127
Triad Women's Project, 43-46
WELL Project, 72-73

Therapy for Adults Molested as Children (Briere), 48

Training, 176-177

Transitions, 157-158

Transportation issues, 153,177

Trauma, 133
central role of, 87

Trauma and Recovery Model of Herman, 167

Trauma-informed services, 52,65,138, 194-195,196-197
PROTOTYPES centers, 87-88

Trauma Liaison, 31

Trauma phase, 27-28

Trauma Recovery and Empowerment (Harris), 48

Trauma Recovery and Empowerment Profile (TREP), 192-194

Trauma-related services, 188-189

Trauma-specific groups, 75

Trauma-specific services, 166-168

Trauma Symptom Checklist, 49

Treating Addicted Survivors of Trauma (Evans & Sullivan), 48

TREM Fidelity Scale, 187-188

TREM groups, 107,187-188
booster, 197

TREM Model, 150-151,167-168, 172-173,181,184-185. *See also* Integrated Trauma Services Teams
attractiveness of, 188
consumer satisfaction with, 188
gender specificity, 189-190
potential risks and benefits, 188
trauma-related service context, 188-189

TREP (Trauma Recovery and Empowerment Profile), 192-194

Triad Specialist model, 49

Triad Women's Project, 41-61
Clinical Interventions Committee, 48-49
Consumer Advisory Board, 55-56
ethnic and cultural studies, 45-46
group therapy, 52-53
integration development, 50-51
intervention descriptions, 51-59
intervention development, 47-50
lessons learned, 58-59
parenting intervention, 57
philosophy and principles, 51-52
problem statement, 42-43
resource coordination and advocacy, 55
target population, 43-46
Wisdom of Women (WOW) peer support group, 56-57

Trust issues, 103

University of Kansas, 169
University of South Florida, 41-61, xiv

Veysey, Bonita M., xiv
Vicarious traumatization, 138
Violence, consequences of, 5-7
Volunteer positions, 32

Welfare reform, 83
WELL Child Project, 65,77
Wellesley College, 64
WELL Project, 63-80
 conclusions, 77-78
 integrated interventions, 74-78
 integration, 67-68
 integration: agency-level, 68-69
 integration: community-level, 69-70
 integration: consumer, 71-72
 integration: existing service, 73-74
 integration: state-level, 70-71
 interagency service planning, 74
 parenting groups, 75-76
 peer-led mutual help groups, 76-77

resource coordination, 73-74
 service delivery, 72-77
 target population, 72-73
 trauma-specific groups, 85
*WELL Project Training Curriculum
 for Providers,* 68
Western Massachusetts Training
 Consortium, 19-39
Wisconsin Quality of Life Instrument,
 49
Wisdom of Women (WOW) peer
 support group, 50,56-57
Women, Co-occurring Disorders and
 Violence Study, 1-18,64
 description, 8-11
 literature review, 4-7
 overview of report, 11-13
 SAMHSA leadership, 7-8
 service system issues, 2-4
Women Embracing Life and Living
 Project, 63-80. *See also*
 WELL Project
Women's Circle residential center, 108
Women's Treatment Specialists,
 128-129,133

BOOK ORDER FORM!

Order a copy of this book with this form or online at:
http://www.haworthpress.com/store/product.asp?sku=5343

Responding to Physical and Sexual Abuse in Women with Alcohol and Other Drug and Mental Disorders
Program Building

___ in softbound at $29.95 (ISBN: 978-0-7890-2604-0)
___ in hardbound at $49.95 (ISBN: 978-0-7890-2603-3)

COST OF BOOKS _____

POSTAGE & HANDLING _____
US: $4.00 for first book & $1.50
for each additional book
Outside US: $5.00 for first book
& $2.00 for each additional book.

SUBTOTAL _____
In Canada: add 7% GST. _____

STATE TAX _____
CA, IL, IN, MN, NJ, NY, OH & SD residents
please add appropriate local sales tax.

FINAL TOTAL _____
If paying in Canadian funds, convert
using the current exchange rate,
UNESCO coupons welcome.

❏ BILL ME LATER:
Bill-me option is good on US/Canada/
Mexico orders only; not good to jobbers,
wholesalers, or subscription agencies.

❏ **Signature** _____

❏ **Payment Enclosed: $** _____

❏ **PLEASE CHARGE TO MY CREDIT CARD:**
❏ Visa ❏ MasterCard ❏ AmEx ❏ Discover
❏ Diner's Club ❏ Eurocard ❏ JCB

Account # _____

Exp Date _____

Signature _____
(Prices in US dollars and subject to change without notice.)

PLEASE PRINT ALL INFORMATION OR ATTACH YOUR BUSINESS CARD

Name

Address

City   State/Province   Zip/Postal Code

Country

Tel   Fax

E-Mail

May we use your e-mail address for confirmations and other types of information? ❏ Yes ❏ No We appreciate receiving
your e-mail address. Haworth would like to e-mail special discount offers to you, as a preferred customer.
We will never share, rent, or exchange your e-mail address. We regard such actions as an invasion of your privacy.
Order From Your **Local Bookstore** or Directly From
The Haworth Press, Inc. 10 Alice Street, Binghamton, New York 13904-1580 • USA
Call Our toll-free number (1-800-429-6784) / Outside US/Canada: (607) 722-5857
Fax: 1-800-895-0582 / Outside US/Canada: (607) 771-0012
E-mail your order to us: orders@haworthpress.com

For orders outside US and Canada, you may wish to order through your local
sales representative, distributor, or bookseller.
For information, see http://haworthpress.com/distributors

(Discounts are available for individual orders in US and Canada only, not booksellers/distributors.)

Please photocopy this form for your personal use.
www.HaworthPress.com

BOF05